Bhumika Pareek
Shiva Chauhan
Vikas Jindal

TREATMENT MODALITIES FOREXCESSIVE GINGIVAL DISPLAY

Bhumika Pareek
Shiva Chauhan
Vikas Jindal

TREATMENT MODALITIES FOREXCESSIVE GINGIVAL DISPLAY

LAP LAMBERT Academic Publishing

Imprint
Any brand names and product names mentioned in this book are subject to trademark, brand or patent protection and are trademarks or registered trademarks of their respective holders. The use of brand names, product names, common names, trade names, product descriptions etc. even without a particular marking in this work is in no way to be construed to mean that such names may be regarded as unrestricted in respect of trademark and brand protection legislation and could thus be used by anyone.

Cover image: www.ingimage.com

Publisher:
LAP LAMBERT Academic Publishing
is a trademark of
Dodo Books Indian Ocean Ltd. and OmniScriptum S.R.L publishing group

120 High Road, East Finchley, London, N2 9ED, United Kingdom
Str. Armeneasca 28/1, office 1, Chisinau MD-2012, Republic of Moldova, Europe
Managing Directors: Ieva Konstantinova, Victoria Ursu
info@omniscriptum.com

Printed at: see last page
ISBN: 978-620-8-42122-9

ACKNOWLEDGEMENT

"Whatever the mind of a man can conceive and believe, it can achieve."

I wish to thank all those who walked besides me and helped me along this journey unceasingly. I would like to thank GOD almighty with whose gracious and plentiful blessings this project was successfully completed

At this moment in time while presenting my library dissertation, when I look back to count on all those good hearts who have directly or indirectly contributed in giving their precious time and impassioning me in connecting all dots of this piece of work in the best possible form, words would not be enough to express my sincere and deepest gratitude towards all of them.

Words fall short in expressing my sincere thanks to my esteemed and revered teacher and guide, Dr. Vikas Jindal, Professor and Head of the Department of Periodontology and Oral Implantology, Himachal Dental College, Sundernagar (H.P.). His invaluable guidance, constant encouragement, and constructive suggestions were vital in the successful completion of this dissertation. Thank you, sir, for your relentless support and dedication.

My sincere gratitude to my teacher Dr. Baljeet Singh, Principal & Professor Department of Periodontology and Oral Implantology ,Himachal Dental College, Sundernagar for lending his continuous guidance throughout. His unfailing support, untiring efforts, unflinching guidance and constant encouragement has enabled me to carry out this work to the best of my capability.

My special words of thanks to Dr. Shiva Chauhan, Reader for being a source of inspiration and for her constant guidance, patient hearing, moral support, endless words of wisdom and deeds of encouragement throughout. I have learnt extensively from her, including how to raise new possibilities, how to regard an old question from a new perspective, how to approach a problem by systematic thinking, data-driven decision making and exploiting serendipity.

My special words of thanks to Dr. Basant Kaur Aulakh, Dr. Abhinav Bhasker, Sr. Lecturer. Their presence in my day-to-day guidance will forever be a part of me and will be a valuable memory to cherish throughout my life. They have always kept an eye on the progress of my work, and gave their precious time whenever and wherever required. Thanks o them for supporting my ideas, helping me think rationally and for lending her unflinching zeal and thorough scrutinization from commencement to culmination of this work.

I am indebited to my seniors Dr. Shakha Pathania, Dr. Rohan Bhatia, for their concern and timely guidance. I am lucky to have my colleagues who are like pillars of strength in all my endeavours. A very special thanks to my colleagues Dr. Ishita Kaushal , Dr.Isha Badyal ,Dr Neeti Sharma ,Dr Keshav Garg, for their constant co-operation and support and a very special thanks to my juniors Dr. Krishan Sushant Kaushal, Dr.Jeevanjot, Dr. Aditi Chandel , Dr. Ankush Chambyal for theirconstant support and help.

"Next to GOD My parents..."

I feel immense gratitude and deep affection for my dearest parents, Mr. Surender Kumar Pareek and Mrs. Shakuntla Devi, my brother, Dr. Tarun Kumar Pareek and his wife Dr. Pallavi Pareek, my sister, Deepika Pareek for their unwavering faith in me. Their love, care, sacrifice, and support allowed me the freedom to pursue my aspirations. They have been my pillars of strength, standing by me through all the highs and lows of life.

It's my fortune to gratefully acknowledge the support of my friends Dr. Suhani Gill, Dr. Tamanna Gandhi, Dr. Priya Bansal and Dr. Shikha Sharma who stood by me during my tough times and reinforced my confidence time and again throughout my work.

I would also like to extend a vote of thanks to the non-teaching staff, Mr. Kamal Lochan, Mr. Sunder Singh for the help they extended during my work. Last but not the least I would like to acknowledge my deep sense of gratitude towards all those brains and hands whose names might have eluded my mind but that had helped in making this dissertation feasible.

Dr. Bhumika Pareek

TABLE OF CONTENTS

INTRODUCTION

Beauty is power; a smile is its sword.

- John Ray

We shall never know all the good that a simple smile can do.

Mother Teresa -

With the society becoming more and more conscious about their esthetics, the job of the periodontists are more challenged to not only treat and maintain the periodontium , but also deliver outstanding esthetics. Since facial expressions and the smile are key components for nonverbal communication, thus the smile has a significant role in the determination of the first impression of a person.[1]

What is a smile?

A smile is a symbol of beauty and well being in our modern society, human facial expression transcending language, culture, race, gender, time and socioeconomic difference. A variety of factors, including tooth form, position, gingival health, gingival tissue levels and presence of scars may influence overall smile esthetics.

According to Husley *"A smile is one of the most effective means by which people convey their emotions"*

An esthetic or pleasing smile is composed of 3 primary components:

a) The teeth,
b) Lip framework,
c) The gingival scaffold.[2]

An ideal esthetic and pleasing smile presents the following characteristics (Fig 1)[3,4]:

1) Minimal gingival exposure,
2) Symmetric display and harmony between the maxillary gingival line and upper lip,
3) Healthy gingival tissue filling the entire interproximal spaces,
4) Harmony between the anterior and posterior segments (gradation principle[5]),
5) Teeth in correct anatomy and proportion (form and position),
6) Proper color and shade of the teeth, and
7) Lower lip parallel to the incisal edges of the maxillary anterior teeth and to the imaginary line going through the contact points of these teeth.

Thus an ideal or an esthetic smile is equally dependent on the gingival display as well as the tooth shape, size, color, position and symmetry; where lips govern the display of the teeth and the gingiva. There have been studies conducted which indicate that the amount of gingival display on smiling is a very crucial factor to smile attractiveness. One such study by Van der Geld et al. concluded that the amount of gingival display was a significant characteristic in a person's own satisfaction with their smile.

A youthful smile is when there is 1-2mm of the gingival margin visible during the smile, while an excessive amount of gingival tissues displayed during smiling is commonly known as *"gummy smile"* or excessive gingival display (EGD). Gingival display of more than 4 mm of gingival is considered by many to be unattractive. It might be one of the several developmental or acquired deformities and conditions that manifest in periodontium as stated by Armitage in 1999.

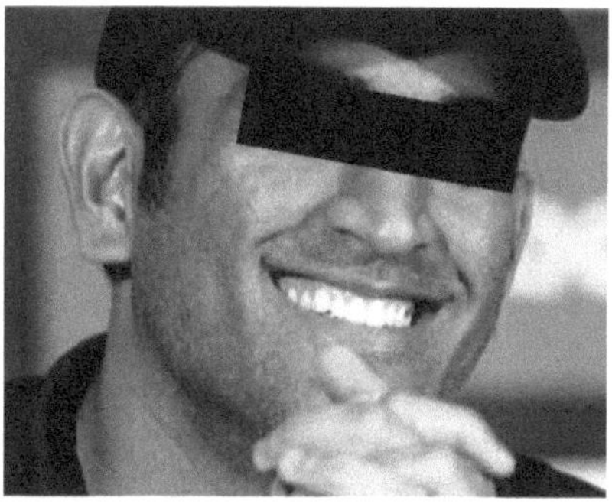

Fig.1.1

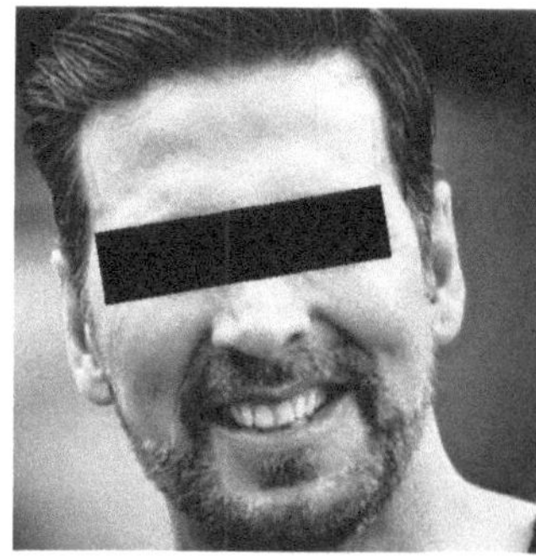

Fig.1.2

Gummy smile being an aesthetic concern , may affect a significant population – Tjan et al. 1984 reported a prevalence of 10.5% & Dong et al. reported prevalence of 29% respectively. The excessive gingival display is more prevalent (Peck et al. 1992, Ackerman & Ackerman 2002) and considered more unaesthetic in females compared to males (Geron & Atalia 2005)

The causes of "gummy smile" (GS) may vary – anterior dento-alveolar extrusion, altered passive eruption (APE), short or hyperactive upper lip, incisal wear, crown length, gingival hyperplasia, vertical maxillary excess, or the combinations of the above as testified by (Graber & Salama 1996)

Similarly with accordance to the etiology, there are several treatment modalities namely implant spacer technique, BOTOX, Myotomy, Lip repositioning, Gingivectomy, crown lengthening procedures, V-Y plasty & lip lengthening procedures that could be employed to achieve the esthetic smile.

Periodontists being considered the oral plastic and cosmetic surgeons, understand the periodontium better and thus can shoulder the responsibility to enrich a gummy smile to an ideal esthetic smile while maintaining the equilibrium between the hard and the soft tissues in the oral cavity.

Some authors cite the characteristics of a perfect smile. Da Silva states that the perfect smile is characterized by exposure of the total length of the upper anterior teeth up to the premolars, showing the incisal curve of these teeth parallel to inner curvature of the lower lip, and slightly touching or leaving a minimum space with the lower lip.

The appearance of gingival tissue also has an important role in the overall aesthetic structure, especially in patients with a medium or high smile line. Harmony of color, texture, shape and architecture of the gingival tissue is extremely important in the aesthetic appearance of the smile. Ideally, the outline of the gingival margin would be parallel to the incisal line and follow the guidance of horizontal reference lines. In addition, it shall provide a suitable scalloped design, with presence of interdental papillae. This ideal contour tends inevitably to change in cases where there is loss of periodontal support.

The dentist should balance the aesthetic needs of the patient with the functional requirements, while harmonically matching the unique characteristics of each individual with the face. A frequent complaint of patients seeking cosmetic dentistry resources relates to dissatisfaction with gum excess exposed during the smile, so-called gingival or gummy smile. The gummy smile is that showing more than 3 mm of gingiva while the "normal" smile shows 2 mm when the upper lip moves apically.

The etiology of gummy smile is related to several factors: changed passive eruption, increased gingival volume due to plaque accumulation or use of drugs and vertical excess of maxilla.

Based on the correct diagnosis, the treatment options are: orthognathic, orthopedic, and/or surgical therapy, depending on the etiology, severity of gingival exposure and the age of the patient. Surgical therapy includes the increase of clinical crown to reduce the amount of gums exposed, increasing the height of the anterior teeth, aiming to follow the contour of the upper lip; requiring, in most cases, a biological space to reestablish osteotomy. The gingivectomy/gingivoplasty can also be used to change the contour of the teeth and their proportions. In association with these therapeutic options, the restorative dentistry contributes by returning the proportion and harmony of the crowns of the teeth, through direct or indirect methods. Understanding the etiology and the treatment options is crucial in the process of treatment of the patient with gummy smile.

Thus, this library dissertation highlights various treatment modalities that can be employed to correct the gummy smile or the excessive gingival display whilst considering the variable long standing etiological factors leading to the establishment of the gummy smile.

CAUSES OF A GUMMY SMILE PRE-TREATMENT

The etiology for the patient to exhibit Gummy smile could be because of:

1. The gingival enlargement
2. Altered/ Delayed passive eruption
3. Anterior dentoalveolar extrusion
4. Vertical Maxillary Excess
5. Short Upper Lip
6. Hyperactive upper lip
7. Asymmetric upper lip
8. Sex predilection
9. Skeletal disharmonies

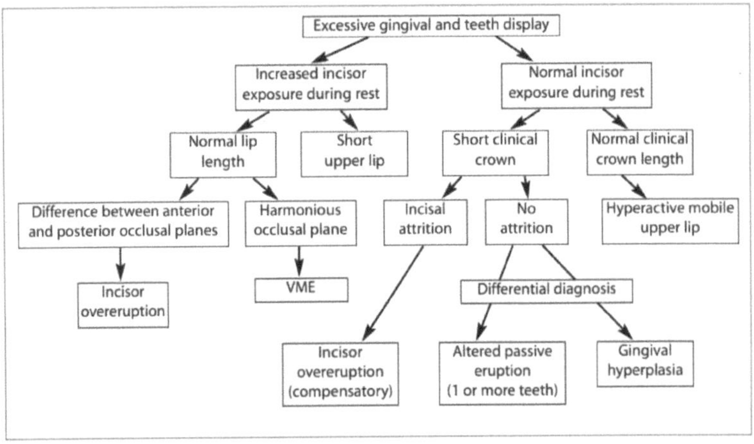

The etiology of excessive gingival display as explained in the form of the above flow chart was given by Silberberg et al.[2]

Several etiological factors have been proposed, which can be pedagogically divided into dental, gingival, bony, and muscular etiology.[6] Figure 3.1 shows a diagram representing the sequence proposed for the evaluation of multifactorial gummy smile. On step 1, the presence of the gummy smile is evaluated. On step 2, a clinical occlusal analysis is performed (overbite). On step 3, a gingival excess is analyzed (a. disproportionate crown width and height and gingival excess). One step 4, the bone structure is examined through cephalometric analysis. On step 5, the muscle analysis is conducted (a) lip length (in lateral pictures); (b) muscle tone (in direct front view). 10

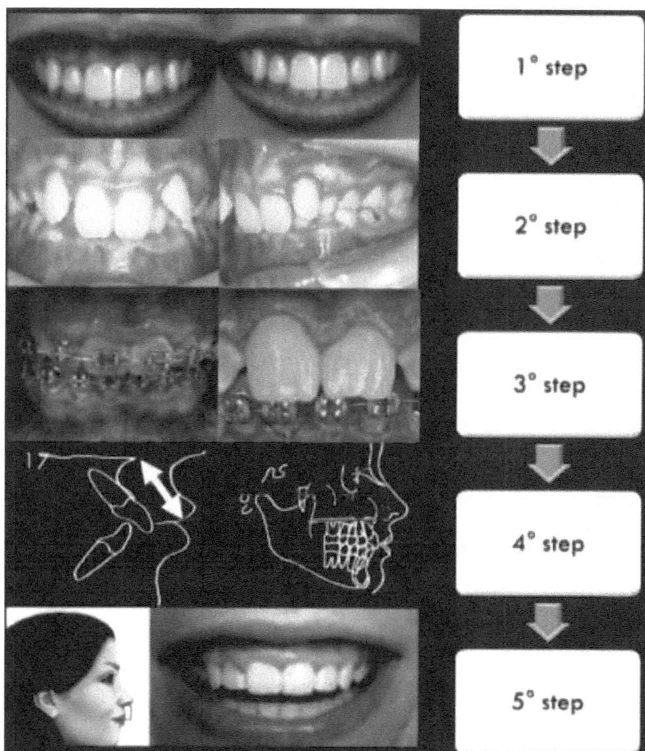

Fig.3.1

Figure 3.1: Schematic representation of the alterations to be observed. Step 1 - Analysis of gingival exposure; Step 2 - Occlusion analysis: overbite presence; Step 3 - Gingival analysis: hyperplasic and passive eruption; Step 4 - Cephalometric analysis: labial relationship (Ricketts analysis factors 17 and 18); bone structure (Ricketts analysis-factors 24 and 25); Step 5 - Muscle analysis – Lip length. (Courtesy of Marcelo Tomás de Oliveira)

❖ SEX PREDILICTION

The gingival smile tends to have a sex predilection. Low lip lines are predominantly prevailing in males by 2.5 to 1 and females show relatively more incidence of a high smile line by 2 to 1 as identified by Tjan, Miller & The.

Peck, Peck and Kataja appraised the observations made by Tjan, Miller and The, and they concluded that at maximum smile, the upper lip relative to the gingival margin of the maxillary central incisor is positioned 1.5mm more superiorly in females than in males. Correspondingly, Vig and Brundo constituted that the maxillary anterior tooth display was approximately twice as often in females than that in males. Van Der Geld and Van Waas further approve the above-mentioned conclusions thereby establishing that the smile line was lower in males and higher in females.

❖ INFLUENCE OF DIMORPHISM AND AGE ON GINGIVAL DISPLAY

The current aesthetic standards establish a dimorphism concept influenced by age and gender. Thus, a healthy and continuous gingival margin display of around 3 mm during natural smile is desirable for females; while in males, only the anterior teeth display is expected, without the continuous band of gingiva. Due to the loss of muscle tone, with a consequent lower visibility of the upper teeth and a tendency to increase lower teeth display, age has its influence over the smile and gingival display.

The lip coverage of the maxillary incisors tends to increase with age, and high smiles will normally diminish with age. Therefore, the gingival smile line may be considered a youthful characteristic. The increased lip coverage of the upper incisors with age improves the smile aesthetics of individuals with gingival smile line while deteriorating the oral aesthetics of intermediate or low smile lines creating less exposure of the incisors and an older appearance. The effect of aging on the lower gingival display is the opposite, with the lower gingival display increasing with age.

Another aspect of the dilemma of treating gingival display is the probable sex difference. According to Van der Geld and Van Waas's literature search, it appears that the smile line was, on average, situated higher among women than among men.

Silvia Geron et al[7] in their study to determine the esthetic perception of men and women to gingival display at smile and speech and to incisal plane tilting concluded that female smile images were scored lower by both male and female evaluators, suggesting that higher oral and dental attractiveness is expected from women than from men. Upper gingival exposure at smile and speech was graded in the esthetic range up to 1 mm. The esthetic range for the lower incisor exposure was with no gingival exposure at all. Images were scored less attractive as the amount of upper and lower gingival display was increased during smile and speech. Incisal plane tilting was graded as unesthetic with above two degrees of deviation from the horizontal in both directions.

❖ LIP LENGTH

The lip length influences the exposure of the gingival display while the patients performs the act of smile. Excessive gingival display is evident in patients with short upper lip. The average length of the maxillary lip is 20 to 22 mm in young adult females and 22 to 24 mm in young adult males.[8] Hypermobility of the upper lip is caused by hyperfunction of the lip elevator muscles[9] and often results in excessive gingival display.

Lip length being one of the vital factors in exhibiting a gingival smile, Peck et al. found no difference in upper lip length between the gingival smile group and reference groups; with both samples having a mean value of 22.3 mm. Schendel et al.[1] reported that patients with vertical maxillary excess had normal lip lengths[2]. On the contrary, in a study by Singer among 70 females portraying gummy smile, Singer found that the gummy smile group actually had a significantly longer lip length than the non-gingival smile samples.[13]

❖ THE GINGIVAL ENLARGEMENT

The smile comprises of lip frame, the teeth and the gingiva. In cases where there is presence of gingival enlargement the crown of the teeth might be disguised as shortened with relation to the increased size of gingiva hence it might be anticipated to be a gummy smile.

Increase in the size of the gingiva is a common feature of gingival disease. Accepted current terminology for this condition is gingival enlargement. The mere growth in the size of the gingival tissues is regarded as the gingival enlargement or gingival overgrowth. The many types of gingival enlargement can be classified according to [1] the etiologic factors and pathologic changes as follows[4]:

I. Inflammatory enlargement

A. Chronic

B. Acute

II. Drug-Induced Enlargement

III. Enlargement associated with systemic diseases

A. Conditional enlargement

1. Pregnancy
2. Puberty
3. Vitamin C deficiency
4. Plasma cell gingivitis
5. Nonspecific conditioned enlargement

B. Systemic disease causing gingival enlargement

1. Leukemia
2. Granulomatous disease (Wegeners granulomatosis, Sarcoidosis, and so on)

IV. Neoplastic enlargement (gingival tumors)

A. Benign tumors

B. Malignant tumors

V. False enlargement

Plaque accumulation on the tooth surface is the most common scenario in the oral cavity. The plaque present on the smooth surfaces like that of the labial aspects or the occlusal aspects has a very low tendency to accumulate plaque and calculus owing to the self-cleansing mechanism of these areas. Thus the most common sites for plaque accumulation are near the cervical region of the teeth near the gingival sulcus since it is not self-cleansed. This plaque on accumulation gets calcified to form calculus which may lead to the irritation of the gingiva and further induce gingival enlargement as a result of this persistent irritation.

In such cases where the teeth and the gingival seemed to be of normal, healthy and pleasing, on such an inflammatory response by the tissue to cope up with the persistent irritation from the calculus, there is the inflammation of the gingiva owing to which the teeth and smile which previously was considered to be normal and pleasing, now appears to be gummy owing to the inflammatory condition of the gingiva, where it appears to be swollen and covered some amount of the clinical crown rendering the tooth to appear small in the vertical dimensions and portraying more of the gingival component while the patient smiles.

I. POSSIBLE CAUSES OF GUMMY SMILE DEVELOPMENT DURING ORTHODONTIC TREATMENT

❖ UNEXPRESSED VERTICAL GROWTH

It is possible that ramus differences are not apparent in children, since rapid skeletal growth, and therefore, significant ramus lengthening had not yet occurred in the preadolescent sample.[15] This might indicate a cause for the skeletal tendency to become gummy during the course of orthodontic treatment and this was advocated in the conclusions that Fields and colleagues asserts drew out of their study.

Orthodontic treatment is often commenced during early adolescence, the growth that occurs in long faced individuals during this time (between childhood and adulthood) appears to convert children with normal ramus lengths and normal anterior dental heights to adults with short mandibular ramus lengths and a tendency toward long anterior dental heights.

This decreased amount of growth of the ramus, appears to affect the mandibular rotation, and therefore produces a steeper mandibular plane angle.[16] Schendel et. al. found short ramus heights in long faced individuals with open bites, but long ramus heights in long faced patients without open bites compared to the norm. Those with short ramus heights and open bites also had much much higher mandibular plane angles (SN-MP) on average (48.61 degrees) than the non-open bite, long-faced individuals with long ramal lengths (39.78 degrees). However, both long faced groups had much greater mandibular plane angles than the norm (31.75 degrees).[12] This finding agrees with the finding of Isaacson et al. who found shorter ramus heights to be characteristic of patients with steep mandibular plane angles.[16]

This lengthening in anterior dental heights (or vertical maxillary excess) that appears to occur as long faced children grow into adulthood, would likely increase the gingival display in these patients during growth even without orthodontic treatment (as previously discussed).

- **EXTRUSIVE FORCES**

The tendency to develop a gingival smile might be improved with careful orthodontic manipulation; however it could easily be exacerbated if not diligently monitored, as many of the forces used in orthodontic treatment are extrusive.

As Fields et al. points out, "although these facial patterns are established early, events may occur during adolescence to magnify or maintain the differences."[15] Because the full effect of this growth pattern is not yet evident during childhood, the prudent orthodontist will recognize this pattern during diagnosis of young patients, and discuss its tendency to produce excessive gingival display with the patient and parents. He/she should also include in his/her treatment steps to control and not exacerbate this tendency.

In a study by Isaacson et al. the extreme variations in vertical facial growth, they state that the vertical growth of the anterior face must be equal in size and timing of the growth increases in the posterior face, or the mandible will rotate at its articulation. According to Isaacson et al., "if the vertical increases at the facial sutures and/or the alveolar process should exceed the vertical increases at the mandibular condyle, the mandible would rotate backward. Conversely, if vertical growth at the condyle should exceed the sum of the vertical growth components at the facial sutures and alveolar processes, the mandible would rotate forward."[16] According to this study, if extrusive orthodontic forces cause vertical growth of the alveolus faster than the condyle is growing vertically, then the mandible could rotate backward even in a patient without previous vertical growth.

❖ ANTERIOR-POSTERIOR POSITION OF THE MAXILLA

With the change in the anterio-posterior position of the maxilla during the growth phase, not only the skeletal components increased in the horizontal dimension as the mandibular plane angle decreased, but the dental components also became more anteriorly situated consequently affecting the smile parameters in the patients.

In their study, Isaacson et al. also found that as the mandibular plane angle (SN-MP) decreased, the mean values for SNA and SNB increased. The mean ANB angle remained relatively constant. The measurements of linear distance from a perpendicular to SN to the maxillary first molar indicated that not only the skeletal components increased in the horizontal dimension as the mandibular plane angle decreased, but the dental components also became more anteriorly situated.[16]

Therefore, Isaacson concluded that the horizontal position of the maxilla effects the mandibular plane angle. For this reason, a person with a forward positioned maxilla and some vertical maxillary excess could have a low mandibular plane angle, and therefore, unless specifically measured, the maxillary excess could perhaps be unapparent upon initial examination. Persons presenting with a forward positioned maxilla whether high or low angle, often have a Class II skeletal and dental pattern. Orthodontic treatment aimed at distalizing the maxilla, or maxillary dentition, to correct the Class II dentition, according to Isaacson's study, would cause downward rotation of the mandible and an increase in the mandibular plane angle, and would therefore allow room for further increase in the height of the maxilla both posteriorly and anteriorly.

According to Schendel and Field's studies, this could cause an increased tendency for gingival display.[13,15]

However, the literature tends to refute this point. In Peck's study, the gingival smile line group had greater values for both overbite and overjet, by 1.5 mm and 1.0 mm respectively. Therefore, it would seem that correcting the overjet, might decrease the gingival smile.[17]

Accordingly, Vig and Brundo found that individuals with moderate to severe Class II malocclusions demonstrated an exceptional resistance to the normal pattern of decreased maxillary incisor show with age.[18] Peck et al. suggest that orthodontic correction of overjet may then improve a gingival smile line in a Class II condition.

II. CAUSES OF A GUMMY SMILE PRE-TREATMENT

❖ SKELETAL DISHARMONIES

Growth of the maxilla is directly related to formation of the gingival smiles.

According to Wilmar, the gingival smile line is often associated with maxillary alveolar overdevelopment or vertical maxillary excess (VME). Peck et al.'s study supports this. They found that the anterior maxillary height (measured from the palatal plane to the upper incisor edge) showed a significant difference between the gingival smile group and the reference group with a difference of +2.3 mm ($p < .001$).[17] In their study of individuals with vertical maxillary excess, Schendel et al. found that all persons in their VME sample, both with open bite and without, showed excessive exposure of the maxillary anterior teeth and poor upper lip to tooth relationships in comparison to the norm.

According to Schendel et al., "extreme clockwise rotation, high angle type, adenoid faces, idiopathic long face, total maxillary alveolar hyperplasia, and vertical maxillary excess all have excessive vertical growth of the maxilla as their common denominator."[12] While many children and adults with long faces also have vertical maxillary excess, Fields et al. found that long faced children did not have a significantly greater anterior dental height than normal children, and while the adults had a tendency for excessive eruption of all teeth, it was not statistically significant. However, patients with long faces do have some characteristic traits, such as increased mandibular plane angles, increased palatal plane to mandibular plane angles, increased ANB angles (and thus retrognathia), and increased lower anterior face heights. Therefore, one might conclude that persons with these characteristics might also have the tendency for excessive gingival display, although not to a predictive level. In a study by McNamara et al, neither the vertical display on smile, nor the amount of upper lip drape was correlated with the skeletal vertical dimension, therefore it appears that vertical maxillary excess is only one contributing factor to a "gummy" smile.[19]

In Schendel et al.'s study, the differences between long faced, open bite and non open bite subjects were investigated. They found that the open bite group had a steeper mandibular plane angle, although both the open bite and non open bite groups' mandibular plane angles were significantly greater than the norm. The occlusal plane angle followed the same trend. The SNA was normal in both groups, suggesting a normal anteroposterior position of the maxilla in relation to the cranial base. However the SNB was significantly decreased in both groups suggesting a retrodisplacement of the mandible. Due to this displacement, the ANB angle was also significantly increased in both groups. Both the posterior height of the maxilla and the anterior dental height were significantly greater than normal. The largest vertical distance between the two groups was the posterior facial height. The open bite group had a normal ramal length while the non-open bite group exhibited a long ramal length.[12] This suggests that there was greater vertical growth of the ascending ramus in the non-open bite group that prevented the development of an open bite.

While Schendel and colleagues found both groups to exhibit an increased amount of maxillary display, it seems evident that orthodontic treatment aimed to close the open bite via anterior extrusion with or without posterior intrusion, would exacerbate this problem. The influence of skeletal disharmonies on the production of a gingival smile line has been debated in the literature.

Singer cites SN-MP and SN-Pal as having characteristic values associated with a gingival smile line, however in Peck et al.'s study, the SN-MP and SN-PP angles were not significantly different between the gingival smile and reference groups.[20] The study by Schendel et al. would refute this finding, as they described all of the VME sample to possess both an excess of gingival display on smiling, and high mandibular plane angle's as well as an increased posterior height of the maxilla.[17]

A study by Fields et al. compared the differences in long faced children and adults as compared to normal and short faced children and adults. They found that long faced, short faced, and normal children all have a similar relationship of the maxilla to the cranial base. The long and short-faced children had a tendency for a smaller SNB angles, and therefore more retrognathic profiles than normal children.

The long-faced children had steep mandibular plane angles while the short-faced children displayed low mandibular plane angles. Measures of the total anterior facial height were significantly different between the groups, however there were no differences evident in posterior total facial height. The differences in the anterior facial height were found to lie within the anterior lower face height, as the measures of the anterior upper facial height were similar among the groups. Upon further examination to determine the cause of this difference, they found no difference in the size of the ramus, but the gonial angles were significantly larger in long-faced children and smaller in short-faced children.

Long-faced children had significantly greater posterior maxillary and mandibular dental heights than normal children. However, surprisingly there was not a significant difference in the anterior upper dental height, although the mean height was larger in the long faced children. As would be expected, short faced children had significantly less anterior upper and lower dental height than normal children.[15]

Similar results were found for the adult groups with a few important differences. Like the children, all groups had similar cranial base configurations with well-related maxillas, the long faced adults tended to be more retrognathic, and the mandibular plane angles indicated significant differences. The posterior total facial heights and the anterior upper face heights were similar for the groups, and the long faced adults had significantly increased lower anterior facial heights. Similar to the children, the long faced adults had normal mandibular body lengths and increased gonial angles, but unlike the children they had a tendency toward short rami and excessive eruption of all teeth.[15]

❖ ALTERED PASSIVE ERUPTION

Eruption to occurs in two phases:

A. Active Eruption

Active eruption is the movement of the tooth down out of the alveolar bone into position on the occlusal/incisal plane.

B. Passive eruption

Passive eruption is the exposure of the crown of the tooth due to apical migration of the gingival tissues.

Short clinical crown heights have also been reported to increase the tendency to produce a gingival smile. Short clinical crown heights can be due to altered passive eruption, inflammation, and gingival enlargement. Active eruption is the movement of the tooth toward the occlusal plane. Passive eruption is the apical migration of the gingival margin. Therefore, altered passive eruption, is the delay in the apical migration of the epithelial attachment toward the root surface of at the CEJ. According to Waldrop, altered passive eruption can cause excessive gingival display.[31] Garber and Salama agree stating, "if the teeth appear to be somewhat short and squat-meaning that the vertical dimension appears to be too short as compared with the horizontal dimension, the gummy smile is probably due to altered passive eruption."[8] However, in Peck's study, the clinical crown height of the two groups was not significantly different.[17]

As Garber and Salama point out, in many cases, a gummy smile may be due to a combination of vertical maxillary excess and altered passive eruption. Altered passive eruption can be classified into two distinct types:

In Type I, there is an excessive amount of gingiva from the free gingival margin to the mucogingival junction.

In Type II, there is a normal amount of gingival as measured from the free gingival margin to the mucogingival junction.

Type I is further subdivided into sub-categories A and B depending on the relationship of the osseous crest to the cemento-enamel junction of the tooth. In subcategory A, the dimension between the osseous crest and the CEJ is greater than 1 mm, and therefore adequate for the insertion of the connective tissue attachment component of the biologic width. In subcategory B, the osseous crest is in close proximity to the cementoenamel junction, therefore adequate space for the connective tissue attachment component of the biologic width is not present, and the connective tissue appears to attach at the same level as the cementoenamel junction. This seems contrary to the biologic width, as the connective tissue attachment must be present, yet cannot attach to the enamel. (Figure 3.1). (CEJ – Cemento enamel junction; BC – Bony crest; MGJ – Mucogingival junction).[21]

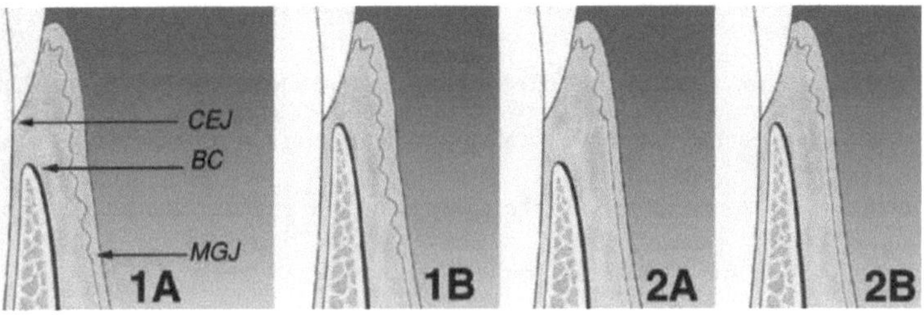

Figure 3.1

According to Garber and Salama, clinical and histological observations suggest that an increased buccolingual dimension of the osseous form allows for apical angulation of the bone crest from the gingival aspect of the periodontal ligament side.[8] While periodontal connective tissue fibers normally run horizontally across the osseous crest extending from the cementum to the gingival, in this form of altered passive eruption, the fibers run apically, parallel to this angular crest, allowing the connective tissue fibers to insert into the cementum just apical to the cementoenamel junction.

The biologic width is approximately 2.7 mm in dimension and is made up of 1 mm of junctional epithelium, 1 mm of connective tissue attachment, and 1 mm of sulcus depth.[13] This "biologic width" is necessary for the health of the periodontium and should not be violated with restorative procedures. Due to its association with this biologic parameter, the type and subcategory of altered passive eruption present will determine the treatment modality.

However, more recently, Konikoff et al. found that 65% of post orthodontic patients had less than ideal length to width ratios in their anterior incisors. Therefore, after thorough oral hygiene instruction, scaling and root planning as needed, and a period of inflammation control, patients with excessive gingival display should be evaluated for altered passive eruption and the need for a periodontal procedure.[13]

❖ MUSCULATURE AND LIP INCOMPETENCE

The musculature can also have an effect on the smile produced by the patient owing to the hyperactivity of the muscles involved to produce a smile.

Peck et al, found that the upper lip in gingival smile subjects elevates superiorly 1 mm more from rest to maximum smile than did a reference group.[17] They also found that the interlabial gap at rest position was much higher on average (6.2mm) for the gingival smile line sample, than the reference sample (3.0 mm). This indicates that lip incompetence can be associated with a gingival smile line. Upon further investigation, they found that 93% of the gingival smile line group were lip incompetent at rest, while only 63% of the reference sample were lip incompetent at rest. When the likelihood ratio was calculated, it was determined that the gingival smile line subjects were 5.5 times more likely to exhibit lip incompetence at rest than the reference population.

In his descriptive essay, Matthews proposes that a person exhibiting an interlabial gap at rest will also have a gingival smile line,[20] however while Peck et al. found that 93% of his gingival smile line subjects also exhibited an interlabial gap at rest, he also found that the opposite was not true. Only 56% of their subjects with interlabial gaps at rest presented a gingival smile line. Therefore, while Peck et al.'s study supports the assertion that an interlabial gap at rest is highly associated with the tendency to have a gingival smile line, it also indicates that an interlabial gap at rest cannot be considered predictive of the gingival smile phenomenon.

Interestingly, Schendel et al. cite a large interlabial distance as a common characteristic of vertical maxillary excess, and these VME subjects also displayed an excessive amount of the maxillary teeth and gingiva upon smiling. These findings suggest that orthodontic techniques that cause lip incompetence might also have a tendency to cause a gingival smile.

CLASSIFICATION

Dentistry needs to formulate a systematic classification to identify various smile patterns. Of paramount significance to our treatment are the terms and classifications that standardize the myriad of individual dental conditions and interpret them into vocabulary that would ease the communication among patients, dentists, staff, laboratory personnel and regulatory bodies.

Despite each individual projects a different smile, three basic smile patterns can be identified. Plastic surgeons, tasked with rehabilitating smiles, have generally identified the following neuromuscular smile patterns: [\4]

1. The *commissure smile*
2. The *cuspid smile*
3. The *complex smile*

Although the basis for smile styles is neuromuscular, individuals can usually employ all smile patterns. Often a smile has been programmed by habit or by an inappropriate positioning of the underlying hard tissues.

Stages of a Smile[5]

There are four stages in a smile cycle:

TABLE 2.1

Stage I	Lips Closed
Stage II	Resting Display
Stage III	Natural Smile (Three-Quarters)
Stage IV	Expanded Smile (Full)

Each and every individual projects a unique smile. Several individuals have a varied discrepancy in their smile lines. In these patients, smile correction can often be restricted to only the maxillary and/or mandibular anterior teeth.[5]

Types of Smiles

There are five variants in smile displayed the gingiva in the smile zone, namely :

TABLE 2.2

Type 1	Maxillary Only
Type 2	Maxillary And Over 3 mm Gingiva
Type 3	Mandibular Only
Type 4	Maxillary And Mandibular
Type 5	Neither Maxillary Nor Mandibular

The above categories are scientifically combined to form a standardization of terms as a nomenclature to describe various smiles. Style, stage and type collectively describe and classify smile. For instance, the most common smile is a commissure smile, stage III, type 1. Examples of each smile pattern with corresponding classification can be seen in Figs. 1, 2 and 3.

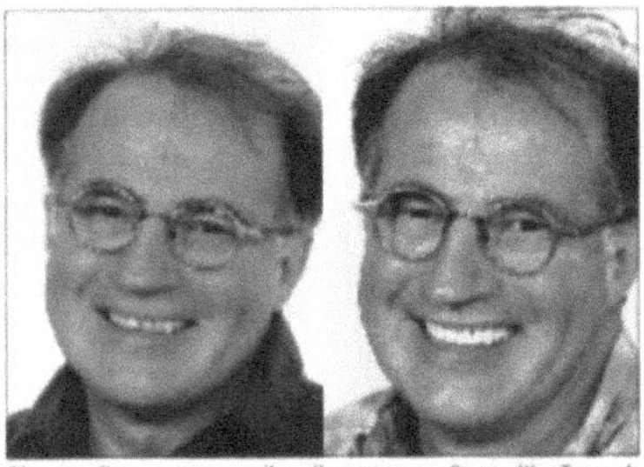

Fig. 1: Preoperative smile: Commissure, Stage III, Type 1. Postoperative: 15 porcelain veneers/crowns: Commissure, Stage IV, Type 1.

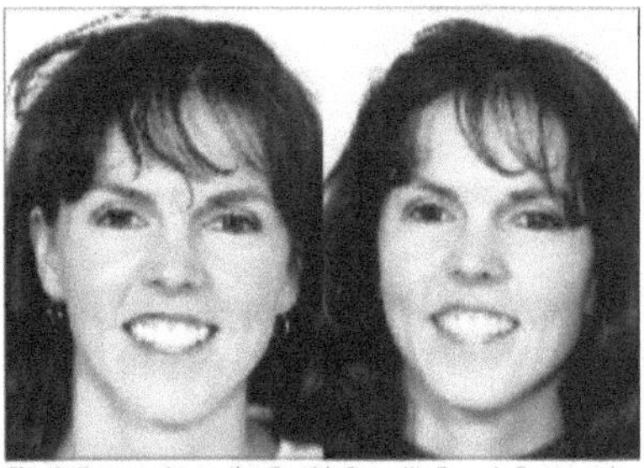

Fig. 2: Preoperative smile: Cuspid, Stage III, Type 4. Postoperative: 6 porcelain veneers: Cuspid, Stage III, Type 4.

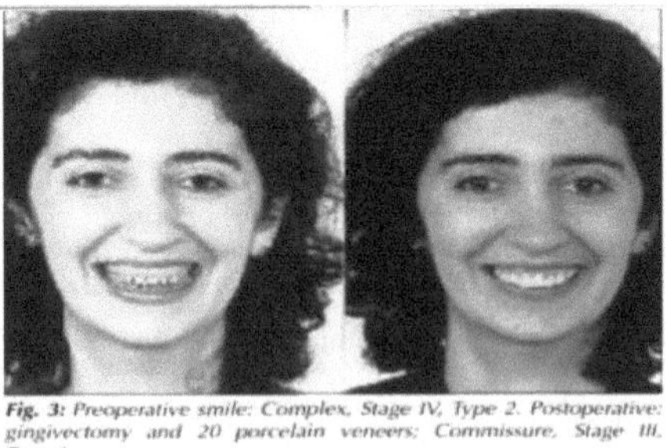

Fig. 3: Preoperative smile: Complex, Stage IV, Type 2. Postoperative: gingivectomy and 20 porcelain veneers: Commissure, Stage III, Type 1.

Tae-Woo Kim et al[6] classified the gummy smile based on the etiology as follows:

- Dento-gingival type
    - Deficient gingival recession, which is revealed by a short clinical crown.
- Muscular type
    - Hyperactivity of the elevator muscle of the upper lip.
- Short upper lip type
    - Short philtrum height.
- Skeletal type
    - Vertical maxillary excess.
    - Maxillary protrusion.
- Dentoalveolar type
    - Excessive vertical growth and/or
    - Protrusion of upper anterior dentoalveolar complex.

Wu et al[7] studied two hundred twenty-eight adolescents with gingival display of more than 2 mm during smile, clustered according to gingival exposure site.

Four distinctive types of gummy smile could be distinguished, and they exposed a continuous band, posterior parts, and one side or anterior part of upper gingiva, respectively.

TABLE 2.3

Type I:	Continuous band of upper gingival display
Type II:	Posterior parts of upper gingival display
Type III:	One side of upper gingival display
Type IV:	Anterior parts of upper gingival display

Garber and Salama classified gingival display and also proposed their respective treatment plan.[8] (Table 2.4)

TABLE 2.4

Degree	Gingival and mucosal display (mm)	Treatment modalities
I	2–4	Orthodontic intrusion
		Orthodontics and periodontics
		Periodontal and restorative therapy
II	4–8	Periodontal and restorative therapy
		Orthognathic surgery (Le Fort I osteotomy)
III	≥ 8	Orthognathic surgery with or without adjunctive periodontal and restorative therapy

Mazzuco and Hexsel sought to classify GS according to the area of gingival exposure and the respective muscles involved. They based their classification so as to perfect the botulinum toxin injection technique for each patient.[9] (Table 2.5)

TABLE 2.5

Type of GS	Clinical appearance	Main muscles involved
Anterior	Major gum exposure (>3 mm) in area between canine teeth	LLSAN
Posterior	Major gum exposure (>3 mm) posterior to canines with normal exposure (<3 mm) in anterior region.	ZM and ZMi
Mixed	Excessive gum exposure in both areas (anterior and posterior)	LLSAN, ZM, and ZMi (combination of ≥ 2)
Asymmetric	Excessive or more apparent gum exposure on one side only	LLSAN and/or ZM/ZMi ipsilateral

GS, Gummy smile; LLSAN, levator labii superioris alaeque nasi; ZM, zygomaticus major; ZMi, zygomaticus minor.

DIAGNOSIS

Diagnosis is the recognition and systematic designation of anomalies; the practical synthesis of the findings, permitting therapy to be planned and indication to be determined, thereby enabling the doctor to act. Numerous observations, individual findings and analyses, which allow a broad based decision to be made for the particular patient, are a prerequisite for a correct diagnosis in periodontics. The information must be objective relevant and accurate.[23]

Two key points must be included during clinical/ photographic examination to determine periodontium visibility. Primarily, the dentist should not only consider the marginal gingiva display (the step before smiling), rather equal significance should be accounted for the gingival display. Secondly, the professional must consider both the natural and forced smiles and the smile lines, when evaluating the position of the smile line in each case.

Thus the diagnosis is further considered under:

A. Intraoral Examination

B. Extraoral Examination

A. Intraoral Examination[24] :

1. Kinetics of Anterior Tooth Display

The kinetics of anterior tooth display is based on the dynamic equilibrium that exists between the static and dynamic states of lip position (Flowchart 4.1). The restorative dentist, when viewing a patient with either inadequacies of tooth length and/or excess gingival exposure, must develop a paradigm for analyzing these esthetic deficiencies. That paradigm must be one that is able to determine if nonsurgical, orthodontic surgical, or some combination of therapies is required to correct these inadequacies. It is far easier and less invasive to correct the situation prosthetically or orthodontically than surgically; therefore, the proper diagnosis is paramount. Spear and colleagues (2006) noted that, historically, treatment began with the biologic and functional basis and often resulted in compromised esthetic results. As a consequence, they believe that when the esthetic requirements are important, they must precede the biologic and functional requirements.

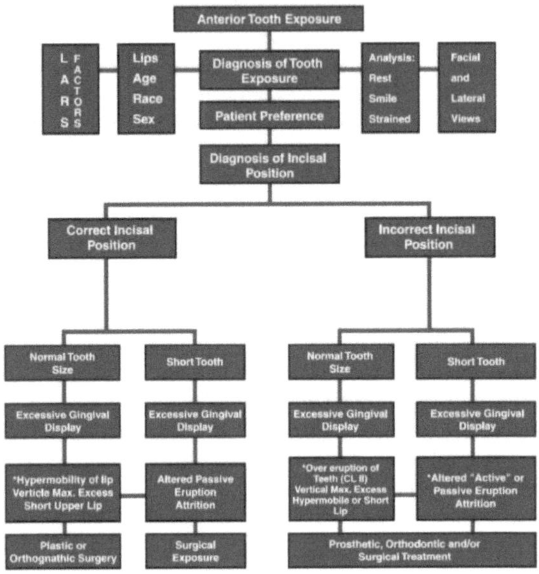

2. Incisal Edge Position

The incisal position of the maxillary central incisor, because it serves to determine the proper tooth proportion and gingival level, is the foundation on which the smile is built (Cliché and Pinault, 1994; Morley and Eubank, 2001; Spear and colleagues, 2006). This is consistent with our previously stated concepts that maxillary incisor dominance and a pleasing width-to-length ratio (0.70–0.80) are the two principal determinants for establishing anterior esthetic harmony, balance, proportion, and radiating symmetry (Ahmad, 1998; Cranham, 1999) (Fig.4.1).

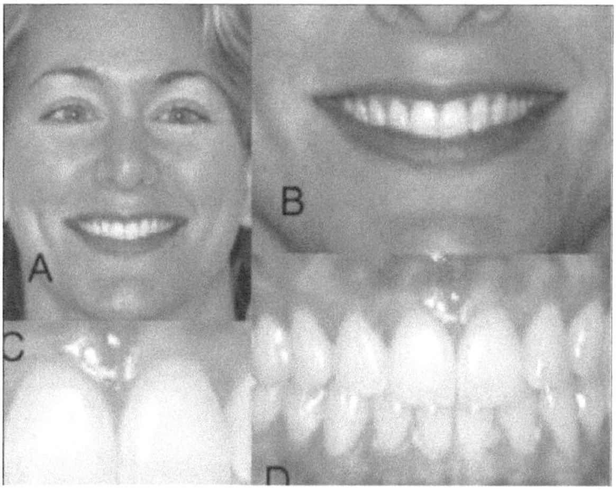

Fig. 4.1. Incisal position and dominance of maxillary central incisors. *A* to *D*, Facial, dentofacial, dentogingival, and dental views showing how maxillary incisal position, dominance, and proportion dominate a smile.

3. Tooth-Lip Interrelationship

A. Static or Rest Position of the Lips.

In the static or rest position, the lips are naturally parted and the teeth are out of occlusion. This has also been referred to as the *M position* (Moskowitz and Nayyor, 1995; Morely and Eubank, 2001) because the true rest position is facilitated by having the patient repeat the letter *M*. Tooth exposure is then carefully evaluated and compared with the expected averages for age, sex, and lip length (Table 4.1).

Table 4.1 Average Maxillary Incisor Display (mm) with Lips at Rest

Sex		*Lip Length*		*Age*	
Men	*Women*	*Short*	*Long*	*Young*	*Middle-aged*
1.91	3.40	3.65	0.59	3.37	1.26

Adapted from Vig and Bruno (1978) and Cliché and Pinault (1994).

B. Dynamic or Smiling Lip Position.

It cannot be stressed enough that smiling is both dynamic and variable and either spontaneous or acquired. The dynamic position is determined by the degree of contraction of the facial muscles, the size and shape of the lips, the size and shape of the dental elements, and the skeletal makeup (Ahmad, 1998) (Fig.4.2).

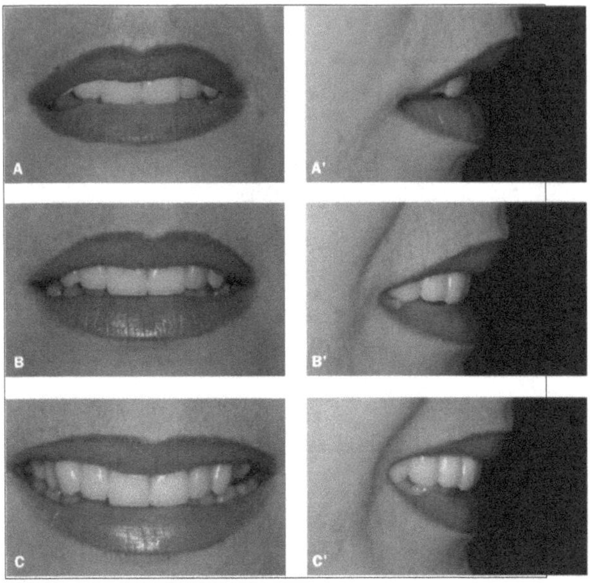

Fig.4.2

4. Occlusal plane

The occlusal plane should be evaluated by comparing it to the anatomic landmarks in the same manner they are accounted during the fabrication of complete dentures. The occlusal plane should closely coincide with the imaginary line connecting the commissures of the lips and two-thirds the height of the Retromolar pad. Considering this approach, during a smile, there is mild exposure of the tips of the mandibular canines and premolars.

5 Harmony of the dental arches

The anterior (incisal part) and posterior segments should be in harmony with one another with a standard overbite and the overjet ranging from 2mm to 4mm.

6 Smile line limits

a) Vertical limit: The degree of gingival exposure ideally should be only 1 to 2 mm above the cervical area of the tooth (Kokich, 1999).

b) Horizontal limit: This is the maximum posterior tooth exposure when the patient is smiling fully both normally and strained. It determines the posterior extent of both the surgery and the prosthetic requirements (Fig.4.3).

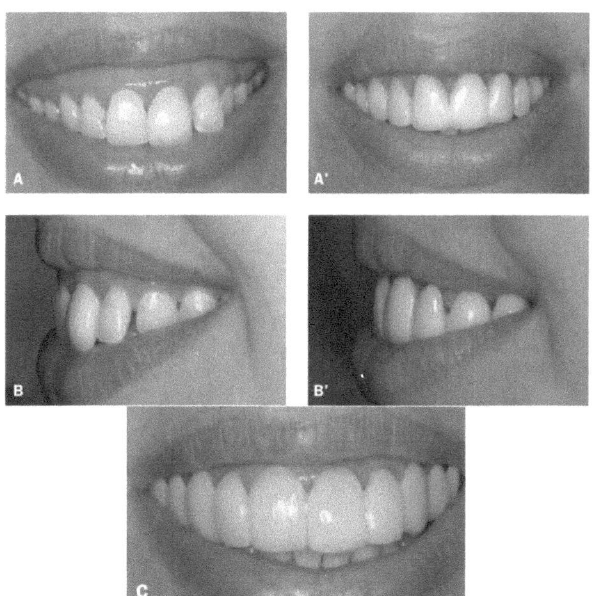

Fig.4.3. Smile limit determinations before treatment dictate the treatment and final results. *A* and *A'*, Vertical limits before and after treatment. *B* and *B'*, Horizontal or lateral limits before and after treatment. *C*, A prosthetic or surgical stent was fabricated to check the requirements prior to treatment

7. Incisal line/lip line convexity:

The incisal line should be parallel to and follow the curvature of the lower lip.

a) Loss of convexity is indicative of attrition.

b) Coverage by the lower lip may indicate extrusion (Fig.4.4).

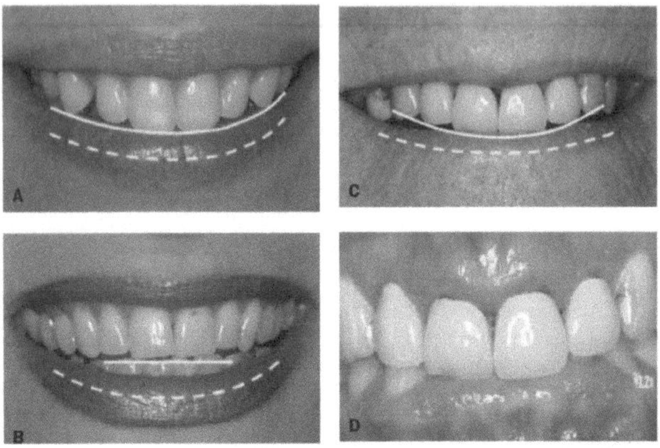

Fig.4.4 Incisal lip convexity. *A* and *B*, Normal and worn (attrition) dentitions. Note the loss of incisal lip parallelism owing to attrition. *C* and *D*, Note the increase in incisal convexity of the teeth with extrusion of the premaxilla, creating a deep overbite.

8. Tooth Size Determination

A. Anatomic Tooth Size Determination. The maxillary central incisor is measured in both width and length and should have the following general anatomic size :

1. Average width of 8.3 to 9.3 mm

2. Average length of 10.4 to 11.2 mm

3. Average width-to-length ratio of 0.75 to 8.0

The clinical and anatomic crowns (exposure of the cementoenamel junction [CEJ) should also be coincident. If not, then probing to the CEJ will reveal the actual tooth size from which a correct width-to-length ratio can be established and acceptability determined. An inability to properly probe the CEJ may indicate a high bone level with a coronally positioned dentogingival complex indicative of altered passive eruption (Kois, 1996).

B. Tooth Size: Occlusal Plane Analysis. Incisalocclusal anterior-posterior plane (IOP) discrepancies, tooth size, and gingival display are important factors for differentiation between overeruption of the premaxilla, attrition, and altered passive eruption:

Robins (1999) noted that excessive gingival display is a descriptive term rather than a diagnosis and requires a differential diagnosis (Fig.4.5).

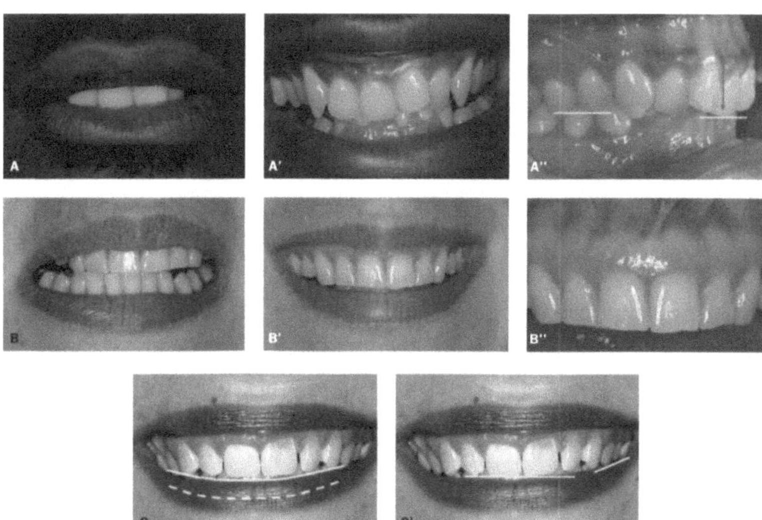

Fig.4.5. Overeruption versus attrition versus altered passive eruption: gummy smile analysis.

A and *A'*, Overeruption of teeth: excessive tooth exposure at rest, incisal convexity exaggerated, incisal-occlusal anterior-posterior plane (IOP) discrepancy.

B and *B'*, Attrition: flat incisal convexity, no IOP discrepancy.

C and *C'*, Altered passive eruption. Incisal convexity normal; no IOP discrepancy.

C. Clinical Crown Length

Assessment of the clinical crown length is a significant factor in diagnosing the etiology of the gummy smile. It may reflect the underlying etiology such as altered passive eruption and over eruption of the pre-maxilla (deep overbite) (IOP discrepancies). Diagnosing the discrepancy between incisal position, IOP, tooth size at the rest and/or smiling positions, and gingival display, are essential determinants of treatment is possible.(Refer fig 4.6)

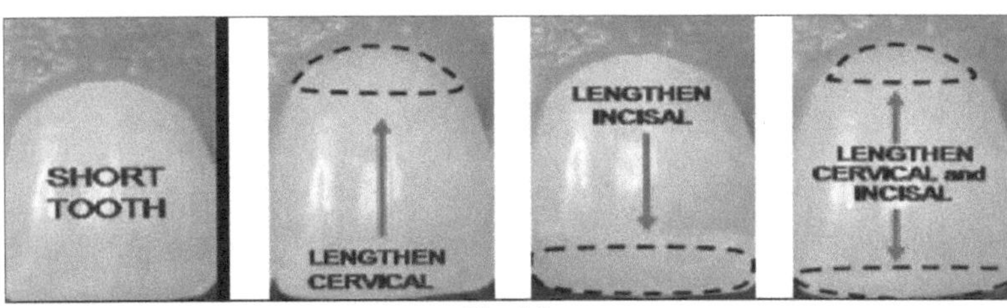

Fig.4.6

Table 4.2 Diagnostic Determinants

Teeth	*Overeruption**	*Attrition*	*Altered Passive Eruption*
Gingival display	Excessive	Excessive	Excessive
CEJ exposed	Yes	Yes	No
Tooth size	Normal	Short	Short
Incisal position	Incorrect	Correct	Correct
Premaxilla eruption	Yes	Yes	No
IOP discrepancy	Discrepancy	Normal	Normal
Incisal convexity	Curved	Flat	Curved
Deep overbite	Yes	No	No

CEJ = cementoenamel junction; IOP = incisal-occlusal anterior-posterior plane.
*Overeruption may result in an anterior convex gingival and incisal contour and the teeth being covered by the lower lip.

B. Extraoral Examination

I. Facial Composition

Frontal View

A. Proportionality (Fig.4.71)

1. VERTICAL DIVISION (Annette and Bergman, 1992a, 1992b; Chiché and Pinault, 1994; Moskowitz and Nayar, 1995; Rifkin, 2000) Using the following four key determinants:

Table 4.3

Tragion (forehead)
Opharic (eyebrows)
Subnasion (nose)
Gonion (chin)

The face is ideally divided into equal thirds:

Table 4.4

Upper	tragion to opharic
Middle	opharic to subnasion
Lower	subnasion to gonion

The lower third of the face is further divided into two unequal parts (Rifkin, 2000):

a) Subnasion to commissures of the lips is equal to one-third or 18 to 20 mm from the subnasion to the upper lip.

b) Commissures of the lips to the gonion is equal to two-thirds or 36 to 40 mm from the lower lip to the gonion

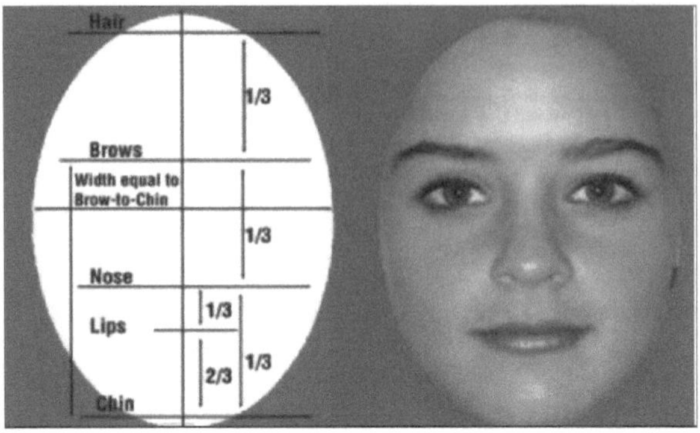

Fig.4.7.Facial proportions. Artistic horizontal and vertical reference lines are established prior to drawing. They permit the interrelationship of the individual parts. The relationship is one that maximizes harmony and symmetry.

Changes in lower third of the face (Arnett and Bergman, 1993) (Figure 4.8)

- Increase lower one-third height
  - a) Vertical maxillary excess
  - b) Class III malocclusion
- Decreased lower one-third height
  - a) Vertical maxillary deficiencies
  - b) Mandibular retrusion bites

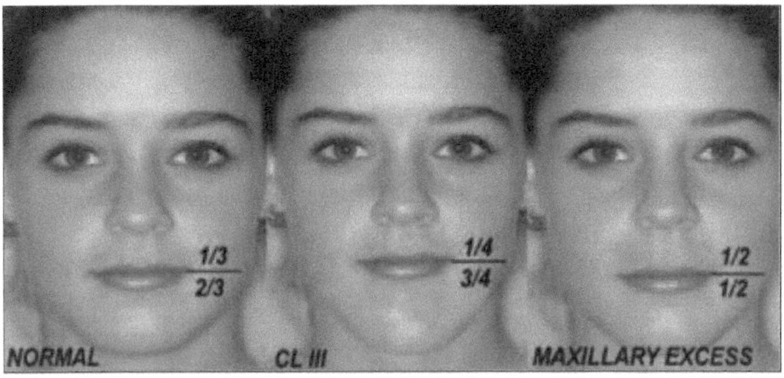

Fig.4.8. Lower face alterations. Changes in the lower third of the face are visualized by changes in the proportions.

2. HORIZONTAL LINES

The key horizontal lines for esthetic evaluation are as follows:

- Interpupillary line (primary)
- Commissural line (primary)
- Opharic line (secondary)

Facial examination

Facial symmetry and proportions in both frontal and lateral views needs to be considered in the form of photographic and clinical examination.

Assessment of facial symmetry is made with respect to the interpupillary line. This horizontal line divides the face into equal halves. Accessory horizontal lines are the ophriac line (a line going through the eyebrows) and the commissural line. These lines should be parallel to the interpupillary line, thus creating an overall harmony of the face. These lines can be used as a reference for orienting the incisal plane, the occlusal plane, and the gingival contour. A line perpendicular to the interpupillary line should divide the face into 2 symmetrical parts.

Face height is usually analyzed by dividing the face into thirds. The middle and lower thirds are more involved in the esthetic consideration of the patient. When measured in repose, these two thirds should be equal.

The lower third can be further divided by the stomion into upper one-third and lower two thirds. (Fig.4.11)

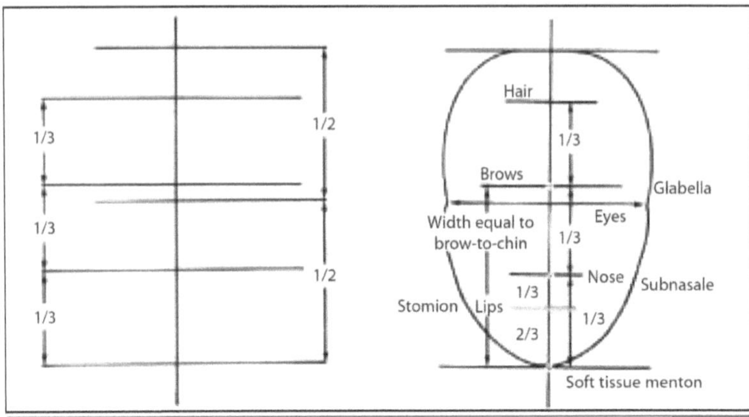
1/3
1/3
1/3
1/2
1/2
Hair
1/3
Brows
Glabella
Width equal to
brow-to-chin
Eyes
1/3
Nose
Subnasale
Stomion
Lips
1/3
2/3
1/3
Soft tissue menton

Fig.4.11

Upper lip length at rest (Fig.4.12)

Upper lip length is measured from the subnasale to the lower border of the upper lip. The average lip length is 20 to 24 mm[13] in young adults and tends to increase with age.

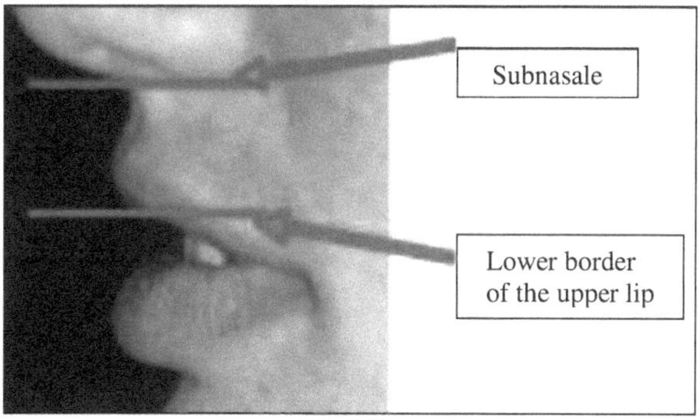

Fig.4.12

Lip length

To assess upper lip length one needs to measure the height of the philtrum and labial commissures. Philtrum height is reflected in the distance between the subnasale (Sn) and Stomion (St) points of the upper lip. In turn, commissure height is obtained by measuring perpendicularly the distance between these structures (C1 and C2) and their projections (C1'and C2') in a horizontal line that joins the two wing bases (Fig.4.13).

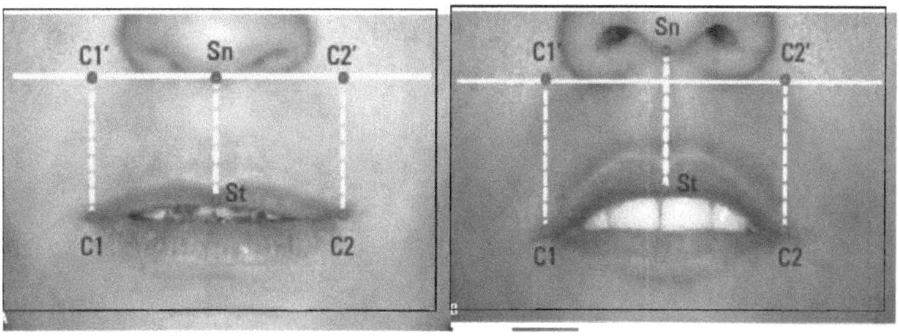

Fig.4.13

The linear values of these measures are not as important as the relationship between the length of the philtrum and commissures.

Thus a meticulous evaluation of the forementioned parameters aids in establishing a proper diagnosis.

ANALYSIS

The gummy exposure could be evaluated clinically and using photometric analysis. These analysis need to be performed during the maximum smiling of the patient in both the frontal and lateral view. With the aim to allow reproducibility of this on a later date, patients are required to smile several times.[26]

It is made sure that all the smile parameters are accurately and precisely recorded during this process, with measurements recorded clinically and photometrically. These parameters have been classified into structural, occlusal and labio-gingival-dental-parameters.

The structural parameter focuses on the facial topology(Fig.5.1): symmetry, face and third inferior vertical dimension and sagittal relationship between maxilla and mandible[24]. Maxillary length measurement in millimeters was done to discover how clockwise rotation or vertical dimension of this structure compromised excessive gingival exposure. This parameter has been measured from subnasal (Sn) point to incisal margin (Incision Ic)

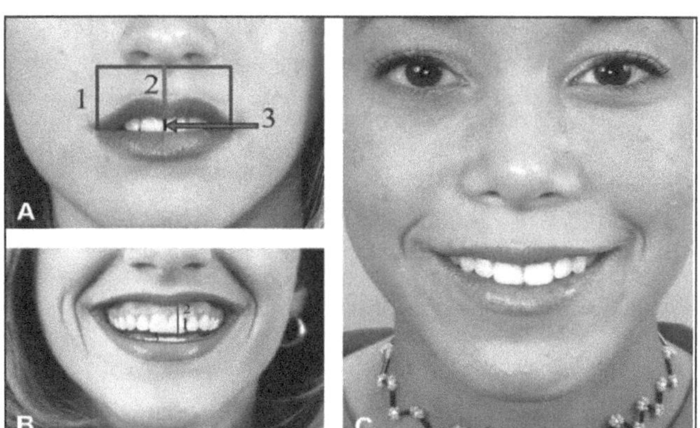

Fig.5.1

The occlusal parameters considers inter incisal relationship ,as the maximum distance in millimeters between mesial-incisive corners of central superior and inferior corresponding incisors, on sagittal segment (overjet) and vertical segment (overbite). Increased overjet and increased overbite was suggested to be associated with the gingival exposure or excessive gingival display. Occlusal plane inclination should be viewed frontally by holding an ice stick in horizontal plane thus exposing the dental asymmetry during the smile. [26]

The third parameter concerned the clinical crown length that could be long, medium and short. It was calculated as the distance between the incisor and the gingival margin. The clinical crown height of the central incisor is supposed to be approximately of 11±2 mm, when it is completely erupted. If the clinical crown height is less than 8mm then it is defined to be short. The tooth inclination is an immediate element in the assessment of the smile.

Labio-gingival-dental parameters considered smile general assessment. The smile accordingly has been classified as low medium and high.

The smile is regarded to be low if the central incisor clinical crown is covered over 1/3rd by the lips, it is considered to be medium if it covers 100% of the crown and 2mm of the gingiva. Correspondingly the smile is believed to be high if it exposes 2-3 mm of gingival

These parameters have been measured during the maximum smiling phase as the distance between upper lip and incisive collar. Another parameter concerning to the upper lip length is calculated as the distance between sub nasal point (Sn) and the upper lip at rest and at maximal smile[26].

The fourth parameter recorded the distance between the upper lip and central incisor margin at rest and at maximal smile (Stomion-Incision Index).(Fig.5.2)

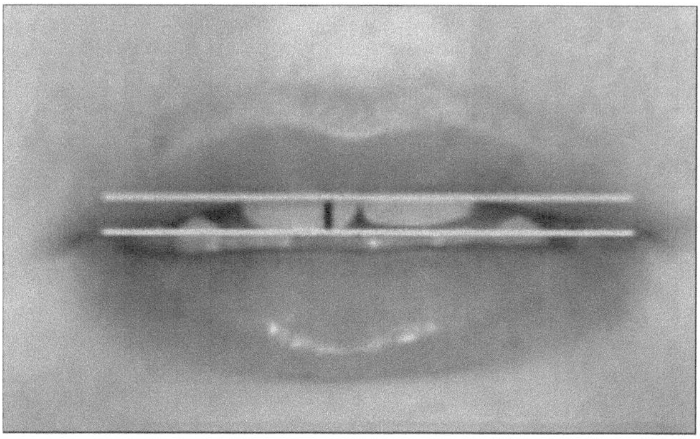

Fig.5.2 Stomion-Incision Index

The last parameter concerned the interlabial gap or the distance between the upper and the lower lips in their resting position and during the maximal smile. Consequently the relationship between the lip and the smile length in these two positions could be beneficial for establishing the nature of the gummy smile. In fact it could be related to the hyperactivity of the upper lip levator muscles or to the short upper lips.[26]

Thus these parameters assist in analyzing the smile of the patient and the possible etiology for the gummy smile and subsequently the treatment could be accordingly planned in each of the cases.

TREATMENT MODALITIES FOR EXCESSIVE GINGIVAL DISPLAY

Ensuring clinical success begins with a careful discussion of the treatment planning, comprehensively covering all possible variables in form of simple to complex cases. Procedures including the periodontal plastic procedures like - crown lengthening surgery, gingivectomy or esthetic gingival recontouring, coronally advanced flap surgery, lip repositioning, muscle resection, anterior nasal spine implant, orthodontic intrusion of the anteriors, orthognathic surgery, Botulinum A toxin treatment and use of several dermal fillers are essential treatment regimens requiring multifaceted expertise.

The interplay of periodontics, orthodontics and restorative dentistry is present at many fronts including the response of the gingival tissue to the Esthetic restorative preparations. Restorations or reformation of the esthetic smile while maintaining the periodontal health are inseparably interrelated. The adaptation of the smile margins or the lip lines, the contours of the lips, the proximal relationship and exposure of the gingiva have a critical biological impact on the smile esthetics and thus a proper treatment planning is advocated in patients with multifactorial gummy smile or excessive display of the gingiva during smiling.

Additive techniques for augmenting gingiva have evolved from the early free gingival grafts through the many different forms of contiguous grafting. This would include pedicle grafts, connective tis sue grafting, semilunar techniques, coronally positioned grafts and guided tissue regeneration [27-36]. Resective techniques involve both the basic gingivectomy with or without gingivoplasty, as well as the full flap procedure incorporating osseous removal for crown lengthening of one or more teeth.

Orthodontic techniques

The great advantage in moving teeth orthodontically is that the entire attachment apparatus, incorporating the osseous structure, periodontal ligaments and the soft tissue components, moves together with the tooth. This means that, in health, during an extrusive movement, the free gingival margin will move coronally at the same distance as the incisal edge moves .Concomitantly, the osseous level will move an identical distance in the same direction. From an aesthetic perspective, this means that any intrusive or extrusive tooth movement can be used to develop symmetry of the gingival margin in a nonsurgical mode. This is particularly useful when any form of restoration is necessary, as a surgical procedure invariably exposes root structure, where the mesiodistal dimension of the tooth is now considerably narrower . In attempting to restore this, it becomes necessary to prepare the tooth and the tissue in such a way that an emergence profile can be developed from deep within the sulcus to avoid lateral horizontal extensions from the preparation line on the narrower root surface to the desired wider form of the restoration. If there is a dramatic diminution of the mesiodistal width of the root at the original gingival level versus the desired level, then orthodontics may be the treatment of choice.

The gummy smile or high lip line case with an expanse of soft tissue can result from two basic problems:

- Altered passive eruption
- Vertical maxillary excess

Thus the treatment of the gummy smile is considered in accordance to the etiological factors associated with the pronounced display of the gingiva during smiling. Considering the vertical maxillary cxccss and altered passive eruption to be the etiology for gummy smile the following treatment modalities could be ideal. (Table 6.1)

Table 6.1 Treatment of the gummy smile: altered passive eruption or vertical maxillary excess

Condition	Treatment options
Altered passive eruption type 1-A	Gingivectomy
Altered passive eruption type 1-B	Flap with osseous resection
Vertical maxillary excess - degree 1	Orthodontics Orthodontics and periodontics Periodontics Periodontics and restorative dentistry
Vertical maxillary excess - degree 2	Periodontics and restorative dentistry Orthognathic surgery
Vertical maxillary excess - degree 3	Orthognathic surgery plus periodontics and restorative dentistry where necessary

These therapeutic alternatives, in accordance with the underlying etiology, are usually multidisciplinary and multifactorial. The following alternatives are presented in the literature:

- Periodontal surgery for cases of excessive gingival display or passive eruption;
- Orthodontic mechanics associated with intrusive mini implants in cases of overbite with extrusion of upper anterior teeth, and additional periodontal surgery to remove excessive gingival tissue and bone volume, resulting from the applied mechanics;
- Surgery of the muscular tissue for cases of short upper lip
- Orthognathic surgery in cases of excessive vertical growth;

- Use of Botox or surgery of the muscular tissue for cases of hypercontraction of elevator muscles of upper lip.

Inter-disciplinary treatment syndicates the aesthetic and the biological principles, as well as periodontal and surgical techniques essential for the accomplishment of a patient's comprehensive treatment. Inter-disciplinary handling of patients is undeniably the best possible professional approach which will elicit favorable results.

GINGIVECTOMY, GINGIVOPLASTY AND MUSCLE RESECTION

Gingivectomy is the excisional removal of the gingival tissue and gingivoplasty is reshaping of the reshaping of the gingiva to attain a more physiologic contour, and muscle resection is the act of incising the muscle fibres[24]

The rationale of combing gingivectomy and muscle resection is to eliminate the pocket, establish a physiologic gingival contour and relieve the forces on the upper lip as a result of hyperactive muscle activity.

In cases where there is more than one etiology, there is an adequate treatment for each kind of etiology, and two or more techniques can be associated.

When gummy smile is caused by excessive gingival tissue partially covering the anatomical crown of the teeth (which is also caused by altered passive eruption), a resective gingival surgery (gingivoplasty) is recommended. Polo, Rubinstein and Kostianovsky describe a procedure in which a portion of the gingival and buccal [3] mucosa is resected and the borders approximated and sutured.[8] Litton and Fournier describe a procedure to detach the elevator muscles from the maxilla,[7] while Miskinyar describes a technique in which he performs a myectomy and partial [3] amputation of the levator labii superioris muscles.[9] However, Ellenbogen reports that resection of the levator labii superioris is short lived, and the gummy smile returns within six months. He suggests placing either a nasal cartilage or prosthetic material as a spacer to prevent this reunion of the muscle fibers and reoccurrence of the gummy smile.[40] Miskinyar reported good results with this technique at 8 year follow ups, but points out possible disadvantages including migration of the spacer to a foreign site, foreign body reaction if a prosthetic implant is used, and the need for a second surgical procedure if nasal cartilage is used.[39]

Rees and LaTrenta describe a camouflage procedure for long faced syndrome patients in which subperiosteal dissection of the lip elevators is performed,[21] and Ezquerra et al. describe a multidisciplinary approach that incorporates lefort osteotomies, with gingival remodeling, and the procedure described by Rees and LaTrenta.[12].

Thus, Storrer et al[41] described a new surgical technique a to position the gingival margin more apically, without exposing the root surface, observing the amount of keratinized gingiva and the relationship between the cemento-enamel junction, the gingival margin and the alveolar bone crest.[5,6] However, some cases are not solved only through gingival recontouring (GR) because the amount of gingival display on smile is still significant thereby proposing the combination of GR + the traction and containment surgery of the elevator muscle of upper lip and wing of nose (EMULWN) can be employed.

Such a technique requires the knowledge of anatomy, location and insertions of the EMULWN. This surgical technique was first demonstrated in a corpse from the Miami Anatomical Research Center (MARC) . This technique is considered a surgical innovation and has not been reported in the scientific literature yet.

Initially, the technique of GR is performed under the effect of an infiltrative infraorbital anesthesia on both sides of the maxilla. The gingival groove is measured and marked in its maximum depths using the krane Kaplan pocket marker or periodontal probe in order to identify the homogeneity of the probing values. Subsequently, a superficial delimitation joining the markings previously prepared is executed with a scalpel blade 15. These markings are deepened with the same blade in an internally beveled incision pattern. In addition, intrasulcular incisions are made in order to remove the gingival tissue that partially covers the anatomical crown of the teeth. A slight elevation of the flap is made with a Molt Periosteal Elevator and the flap is kept in the keratinized gingiva in order to loosen the fibers and avoid the recurrence or regrowth of the gingival margins on the crown of the teeth. The apical part of the gingiva is preserved in order to support the sutures, which will contain the elevator muscle of upper lip and wing of nose. Some suspensory sutures are made after the repositioning of the flap (Fig.6.2.1-6.2.6)

Subsequently, a vertical incision is made on the labial frenum and two more horizontal incisions are made on the mucogingival junction, starting from the frenum up to the height of the canines. The flap is carefully divulged with Goldman Fox scissors and also a curved hemostat, separating the external epithelium from the muscle bundle mucosa, on both sides, at the height of the lateral incisors and canines. With an absorbable suture thread, the elevator muscle of upper lip and wing of nose is pulled downwards, repositioning its bundle adjacent to the highest portion of the keratinized gingiva. Simple sutures are placed, as many as necessary, in order to contain the pulled muscle in this position, followed by the continuous sutures in the labial frenum.

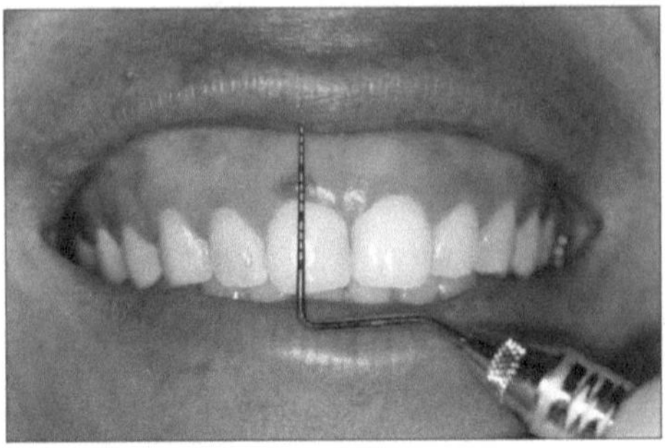

Fig.6.2.1 Measurement of the gummy smile, with the help of a periodontal probe, with 7 mm of gingival display

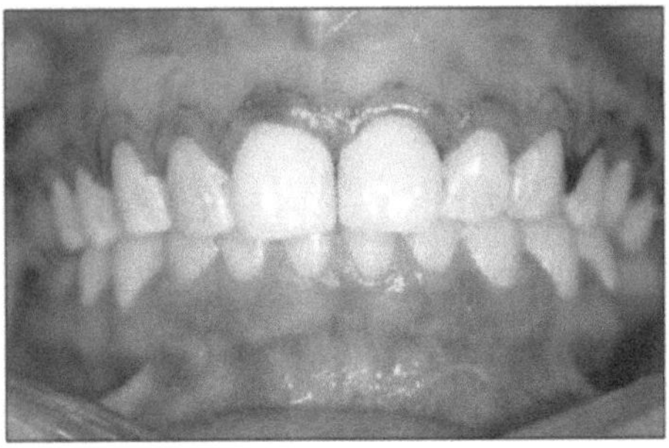

Fig.6.2.2 Markings of the depth of gingival sulcus with a periodontal probe or a Crane Kaplan probe. Union of these markings with an internal bevel incision

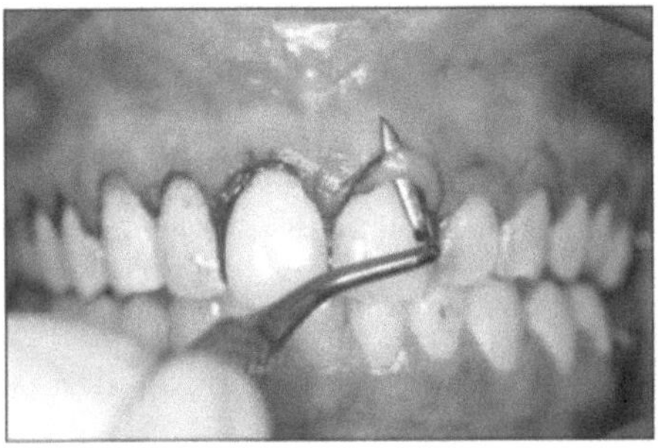

Fig.6.2.3 The excess of gingival tissue is removed with the use of an Orban knife. Note the significant increase of the dental crowns

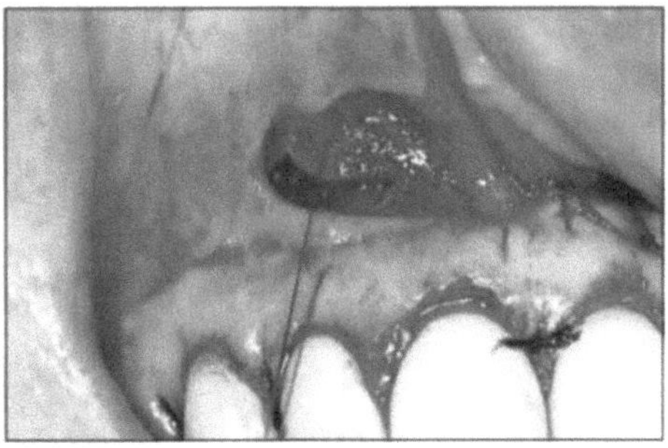

Fig.6.2.4 Traction of the elevator muscle of the upper lip and wing of nose with an absorbable suture thread. Sutures in a deep layer between the muscle and the upper portion of the keratinized gingiva

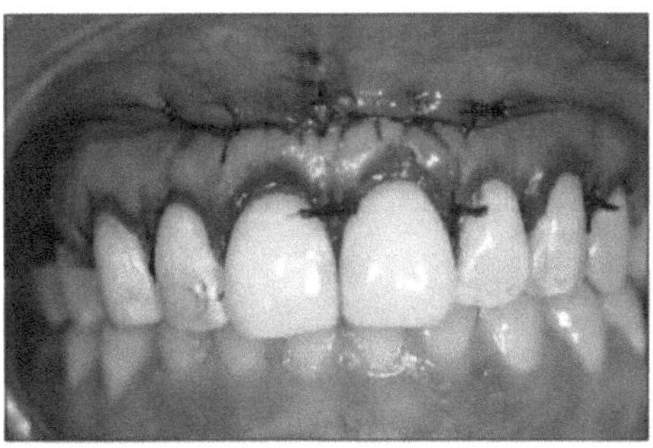

Fig.6.2.5 Continuous suture made with a 4-0 silk thread on the labial frenum and in between the mucosa and the keratinized gingiva

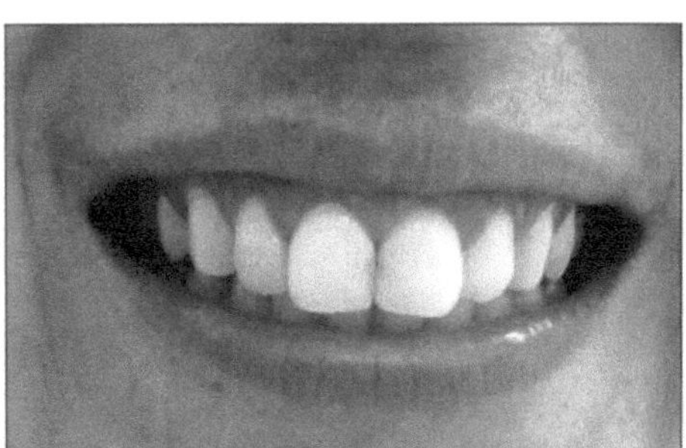

Fig.6.2.6 The patient's lip was repositioned closer to the teeth. It was brought down to show less gingiva

ANTERIOR NASAL SPINE IMPLANTS

The concept of anterior nasal spine implants was first introduced by Mario Polo (2015) [55] and is presently a procedure that is often advocated in case signifying hypermobility of the upper lip as the etiology for the gummy smile where the upper lips are stabilized to achieve an esthetic smile

Subsequently, in addition to surgical resection of the elevator muscles and botulinium toxin to reduce the activity of the muscles, the use of an anterior nasal spine implant has been reported to mechanically obstruct the lip from raising and thus reduce the amount of gingiva displayed upon smiling. Austin describes a technique in which a pouch is created by elevating the periosteum from the anterior nasal spine and adjacent maxilla for 10 mm on each side. It is then filled with a silicone implant material, which is allowed to harden and conform to shape of the area. It is then removed, trimmed to prevent protuberant edges and then reimplanted into the pouch and the pocket is sutured. He reports excellent results and pleased patients with a mean follow up of three years. He reports only one infection requiring removal of the implant and suggests both IV and local antibiotics to prevent this complication.

A technique where cartilage or ePTFE implants are placed between the medial crura of the lateral nasal cartilages and sutured to the nasal septum. Thus the lack of support of the upper lip subjected to elevation by the muscles involved in production of the smile i.e. Levator Labii Superioris Alaeque Nasi, Levator Labia Superioris, Zygomaticus Major, Zygomaticus Minor, and Depressor Septi Nasi (DSN) – are controlled by the augmentation of the septum inferiorly at the midline. This apparent lack of support while these muscles contract when smiling could account for the so-called Hypermobile lip or short upper lip leading to excessive display of the gingiva while smiling.

The cartilaginous augmentation of the nasal septum produces an autogenous barrier, which could block and limit the amount of the elevation of the upper lips while the lip elevators continue executing their usual contraction rate. On the contrary when the BOTOX injections are used for chemodenervation and therapeutic corrections of the excessive gingival display, lip elevator muscle contraction is blocked.

The measurement of columella upward maximum movement (CUMM) plays a significant role in evaluating the need for this grafting procedure, or any other procedure under consideration by the clinician.

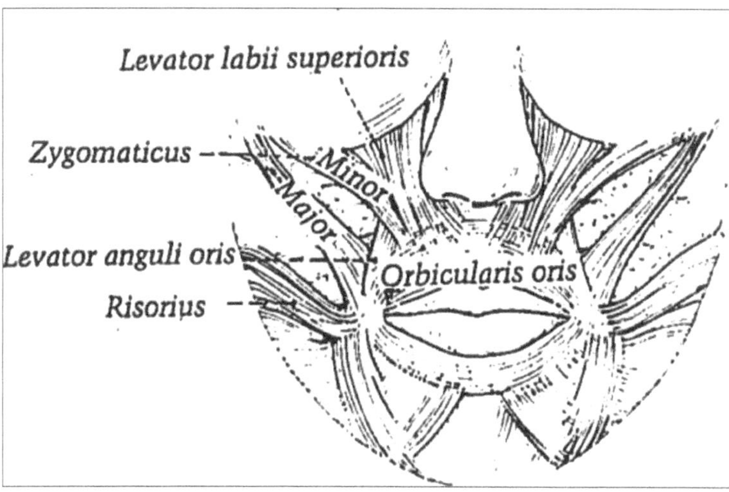

Fig.6.4.1

Fig.6.4.1 The muscles of the smile –the elevator (levator labii superioris, Zygomaticus minor, and levator Anguli Oris), and the spreaders (Zygomaticus major and Risorius) – are seen in their normal anatomical positions inserting into the Orbicularis Oris.

The small septal and alar depressions (Nasalis and Depressor Septi Nasi) have no effect on the lip and are not llustrated.[56]

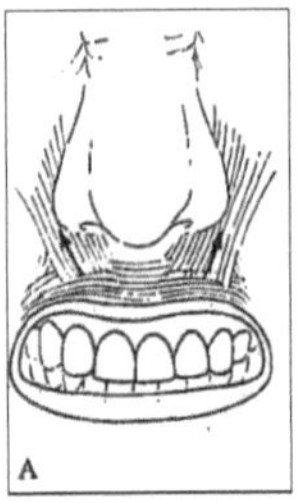

A. Contractions of the elevators (as in winking the nose) shows the gums above the central incisors. This movement isolates the elevators from the spreaders.

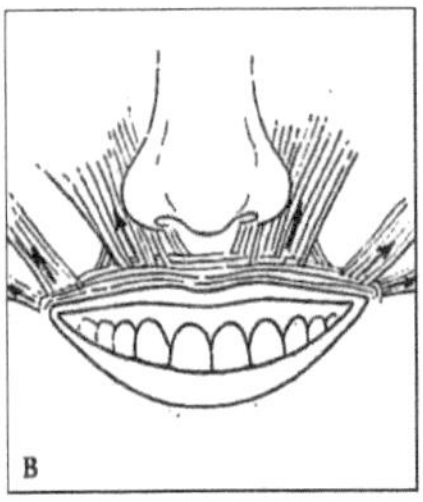

B. Adding the actions of the elevators in a smile, it can be seen that the gumminess is related to the excursion of the elevators.

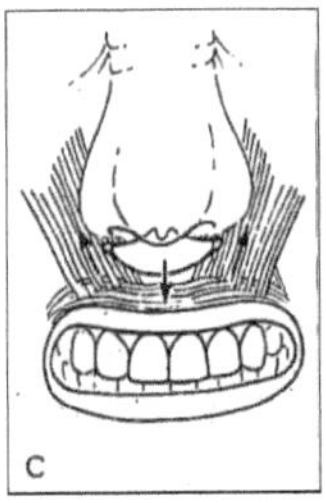

C. Insertion of the silicone spacer implant after partial transection of the major elevators (levator labii superioris) decreases the excursion of the elevators thus eliminating the gumminess

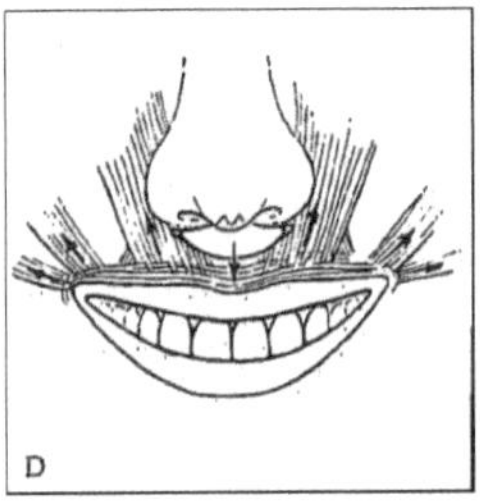

D. When the spreaders are brought into action, the gummy smile itself is corrected.

Fig.6.4.2 A-D

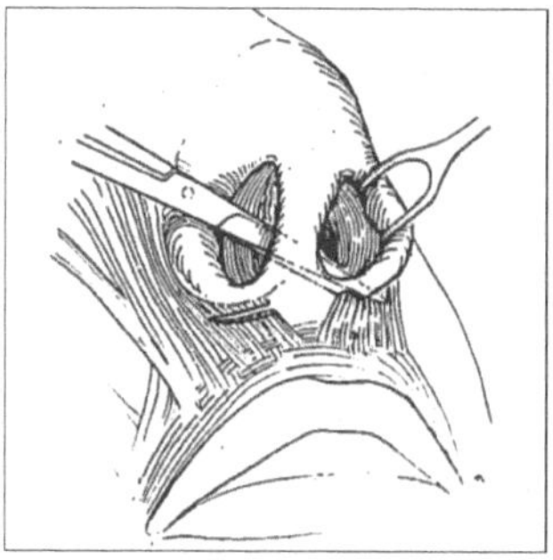

Fig.6.4.3

Fig.6.4.3 An incision is made from mid columella to the base of the nostril. The lavetor labii superioris is partially transected as far as laterally as the ala extends.

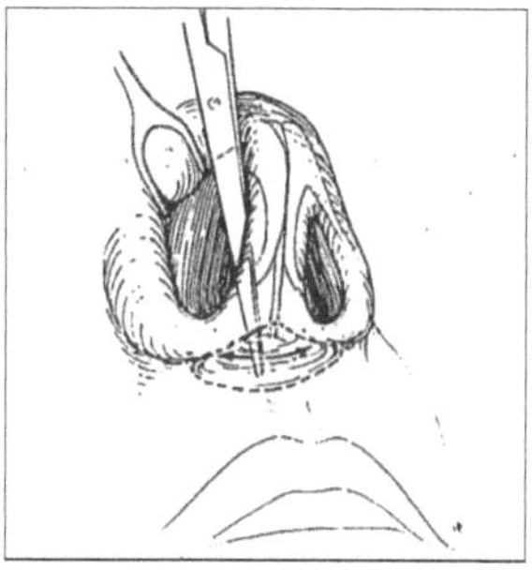

Fig.6.4.4

Fig.6.4.4. A pocket is made between the ends of the muscles for the insertion of the spacer implant, which will decrease the excursion in the upward direction of the levator.

ORTHOGNATHIC SURGERY

In the adults with gummy smile, correction of the smile by several growth modification treatment options cannot be considered owing to the absence of the growth spurts in adulthood. Therefore treatment modality like intrusion of the anteriors is considered for correction of the gummy smile. In cases where there is absence of deep bite, intrusion of the anteriors cannot be performed since it may lead to creation of the reverse smile arc and might even result in anterior open bite.

Therefore, Orthognathic surgery to impact the maxilla is the only true corrective treatment option. In case, when altered passive eruption in combination with the maxillary hyperplasia is present, Graber et al. directs to access and achieve a proper diagnosis of the severity of the vertical maxillary excess and ruling out of the superimposition of the altered passive eruption in combination with maxillary hyperplasia. And in cases if there is superimposition, they state that the altered passive eruption should be treated first to develop a normal tooth form before a final treatment plan is determined.[8] The true severity of hyperplasia can only then be assessed in true sense.

In some cases, the translation of the upper lip from rest to maximum smile is greater than normal length of the tooth crown. In these cases, the patient needs to determine if an increased length of the crown of the maxillary incisors is preferred or some amount of the gingival display. This will prevent overimpaction of the maxilla, which results in burying of the incisal edge beyond the vermillion border of the lips resulting in drastically aged appearance. As a result of which, it is critical to teat to the position of the lips at rest. A minimum of 2 mm of the incisal edge of the maxillary incisors should be displayed at rest.[8]

Peck advocates the surgical repositioning of the maxilla to reduce vertical maxillary excess as the most effective treatment modality. However, he points out to the shortcoming of this procedure – lip shortening that occurs with skeletal intrusion (50% skeletal intrusion). [17]

Suma et al[5] described a surgical technique in a 32 year female patient with vertical maxillary excess. The technique included extraction of all first premolars, mandibular subapical osteotomy to intrude the lower anteriors and correct the excessive curve of spee and maxillary superior repositioning along with anterior segmental osteotomy to setback the anterior segment.(Fig.6.5.1-6.5.2)

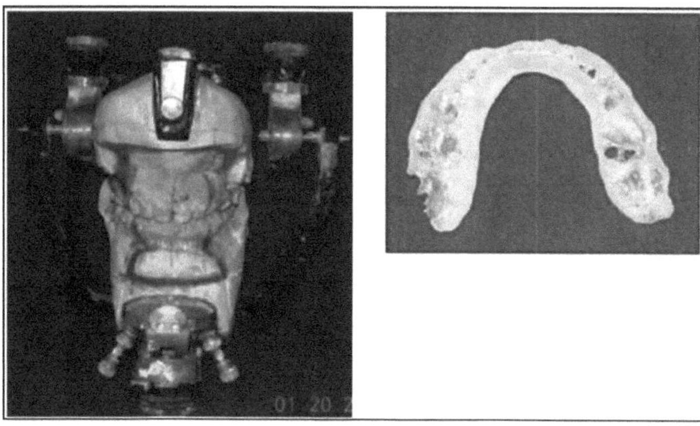

Fig.6.5.1

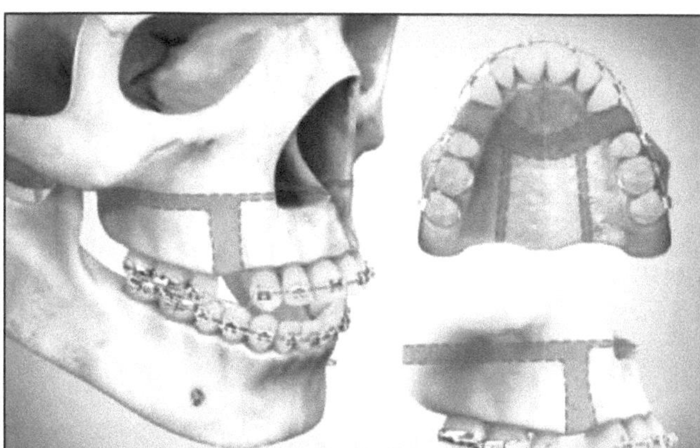

Fig.6.5.2

Pure maxillary impaction surgeries such as LeFort I impaction procedures may also be performed in patients with vertical maxillary excess to reduce the gummy smile. (Fig.6.5.3-6.5.4)

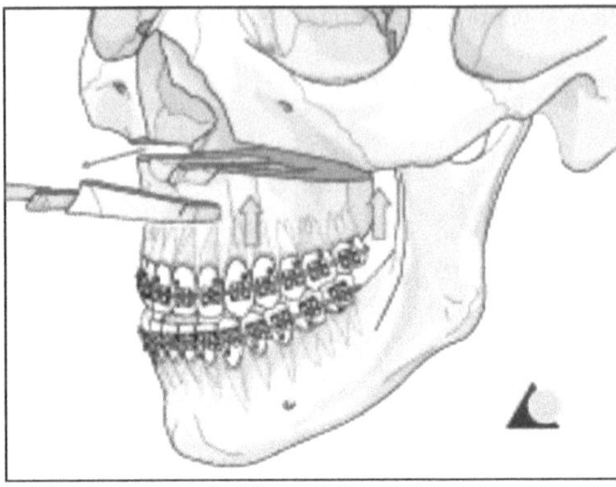

Fig.6.5..3

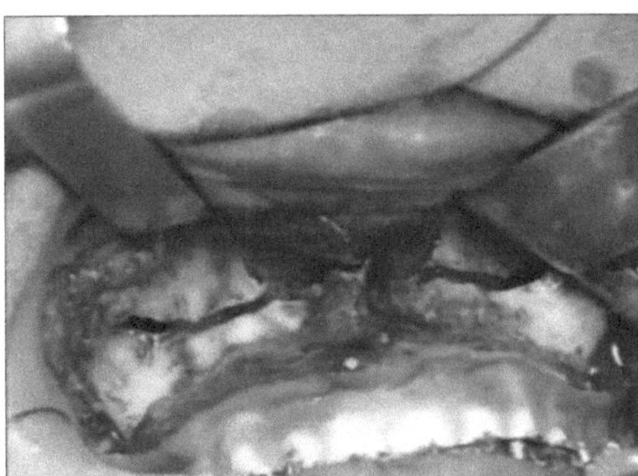

Fig.6.5.4

ORTHODONTIC MINI IMPLANT SCREWS

The concept of correction of deep overbite and resultant gummy smile was fist given by[5] Creekmore and Eklund[7] using a metal mini-implant. They placed a vitalium screw below the anterior nasal spine and stretched an elastic as far as the upper central incisors. They succeeded in intruding these teeth by 6 mm and tipped them 25°

buccally avoiding infection, pain or other screw-related complications. However, the authors considered that it would be premature to disseminate the use of this technique. Kanomi[58] reported that the intrusion of lower incisors in a patient with deep overbite was achieved by means of a screw measuring 6 mm in length and 1.2 mm in diameter. Ohnishi et al[59] also showed a clinical case with deep overbite treated using mini-implants for intrusion of the upper incisors. Intrusion also improved the patients' gingival smile. The effects of mini-implant intrusive biomechanics are still poorly understood.

Currently, the available literature consists mainly of clinical case reports and a handful of studies on animals. The literature clearly shows that teeth can be intruded successfully using mini-screws as anchorage but there is great variability regarding the amount of intrusion, load time, intrusive forces and their relation to root resorption, hindering its clinical application by orthodontists.[57,60,61]

Cases with excessive vertical growth of upper anterior dentoalveolar complex usually show extrusion and retroclination of upper incisors, deep overbite, and gummy smile (Fig.6.6.1). This kind of case could be treated well with the Burstone's Segmented Arch Technique. It would be used "one-piece intrusion arch" for the retroclined and extruded upper incisors (Fig.6.6.2). In this technique, high-pull headgear and precision lingual arch are used to counteract the adverse reactions like extrusion of upper molars. But the mini-implants mechanics (Fig.6.6.3) can treat the retroclined and extruded incisors very efficiently without an extrusion of upper molars and it does not need the patient's cooperation. This mini-implant technique was modifed from the method reported by Creekmore and Eklund[57] (Fig.6.6.3)

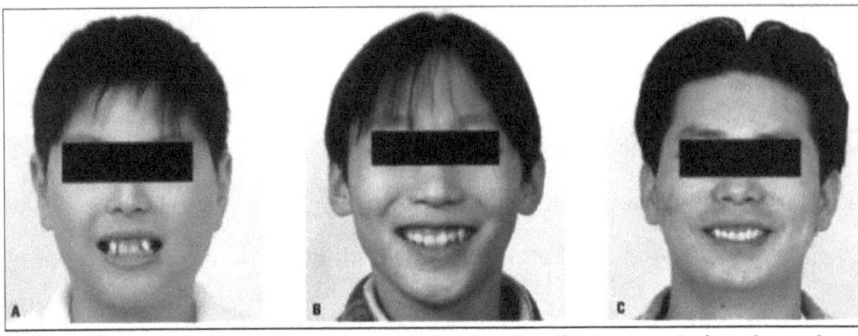

Fig.6.6.1Cases showing excessive vertical growth of upper anterior dentoalveolar complex.

A. Case 1 (10y 6m/ male, Class II, div 2).

B. Case 2 (12y, male Class I).

C. Case 3 (26y 5m, male/ Class II div. 2)

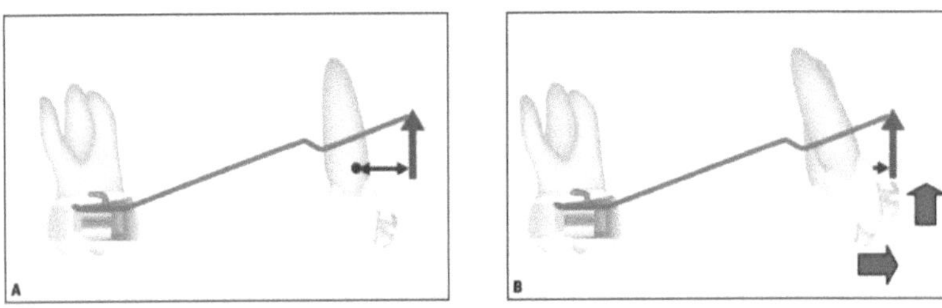

Fig.6.6.2

A. Burstone's one-piece intrusion arch.

B. One-piece intrusion arch is very efficient to intrude and procline the retroclined and extruded incisors without extruding molars.

After placing a 1.6 x 6.0 mm mini-implant without drilling, a NiTi closed coil spring is applied immediately over a 0.019 x 0.025-in stainless steel box wire (Fig.6.6.3). The mini-implant and the upper portion of NiTi closed coil spring is covered by a flap. The covered mini-implant does not cause discomfort to patients and it is preferred to a headgear and a lingual or transpalatal arch.

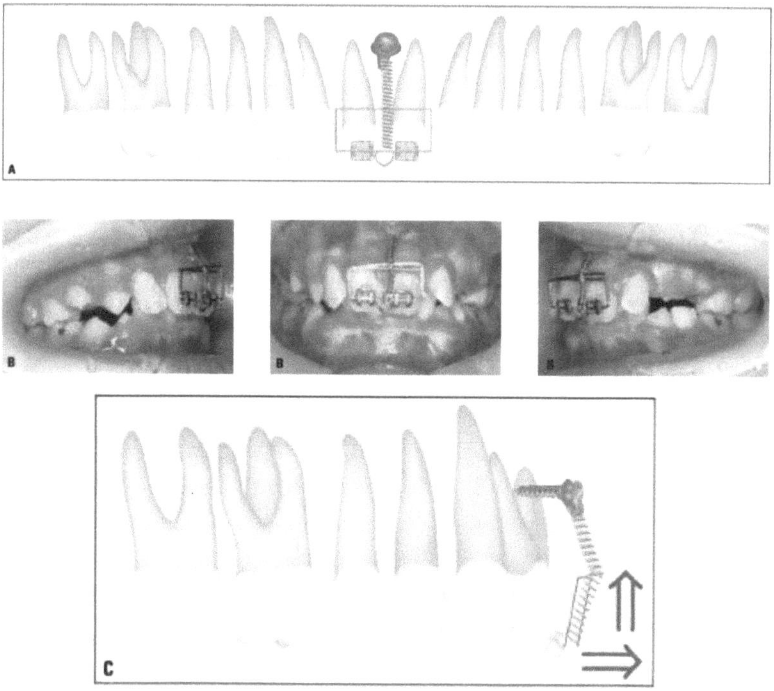

Fig.6.6.3

A) 1.6 x 6.0 mm mini-implant and NiTi closed coil spring to intrude and procline the retroclined extruded incisors. B) Intraoral photos of Case 1. C) Upper central incisors intruded and proclined as one-piece intrusion arch made with 0.019 x 0.025-in stainless steel box wire was used to prevent impingement of gingival tissue.

The patients with dentoalveolar gingival smile are treated with a sectional arch on the anterior teeth, which are connected to a mini-implant inserted between the incisors by means of a closed NiTi spring. This procedure provides some advantages such as no subsequent extrusion, which can lead to a rotation of the mandible in a clockwise direction, opening the mandibular plane and worsening the patient's pattern. This procedure provides some advantages such as no subsequent extrusion, which can lead to a rotation of the mandible in a clockwise direction, opening the mandibular plane and worsening the patient's pattern.

The use of mini-implants in the anterior region was effective for the intrusion of upper incisors and therefore the gingival smile was corrected in all cases. These intrusion movements were obtained easily and without patient compliance. Patients did not complain of discomfort caused by the mini-implants. Mini-implants can be successfully used as anchorage for the intrusion of anterior teeth

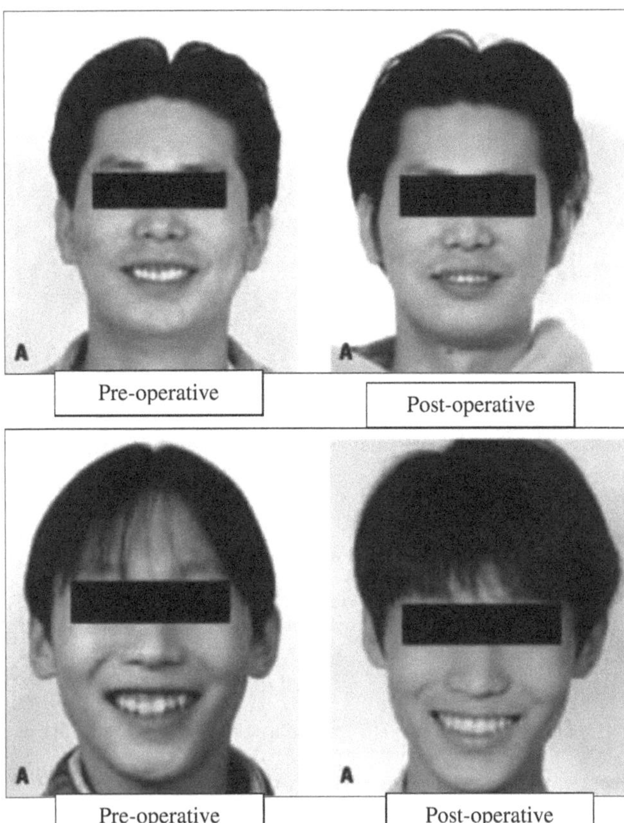

Fig.6.6.4

BOTOX

Gummy smile as discussed earlier could be corrected by several treatment modalities namely gingivoplasty, orthodontic procedures, orthognathic surgery or bone resection. These are highly complex procedures involving moderate to severe morbidity, high cost, and considerable time. This is where the use of Botulinum toxin proposes a simple fast and effective method for correction of the gummy smile.

Botulinum toxin acts by cleaving the synaptosomal-associated protein (SNAP-25) and inhibiting the release of acetylcholine, thus preventing muscle contraction. Among the seven serologically distinct types of botulinum neurotoxin, type A (BTX-A) appears to be the most potent and is most often used clinically.

BTX-A has been under clinical investigation since late 1970s for the treatment of several conditions associated with excessive muscle contraction.[62] Produced by the anaerobic bacterium *C botulinum,* [63] there are 7 serotypes of BTX. BTX-A is the most potent and the most commonly used clinically type. Botox is a purified BTX-A isolated from the fermentation of *C botulinum.* It is a stable, sterile, vacuum-dried powder that is diluted with saline solution without preservatives. BTX-A blocks neuromuscular transmission by binding to acceptor sites on motor or sympathetic nerve terminals, thus inhibits the release of acetylcholine. This inhibition occurs as the neurotoxin cleaves SNAP- 25, a protein integral to the successful docking and release of acetylcholine from vesicles in nerve endings.

When injected intramuscularly at therapeutic doses, BTX-A produces partial chemical denervation of the muscle,resulting in localized reduction in muscle activity. [63,64] Botox has been approved by the Food and Drug Administration as a safe and effective therapy for blepharospasm, strabismus, cervical dystonia, and hemifacial spasm since 1989; in 2002, it received approval for the treatment of glabellar lines associated with corrugator and procerus muscle activity, and, in 2004, approval was obtained for the treatment of primary axillary hyperhidrosis. The National Institutes of Health Consensus Conference of 1990 also included it as a safe and effective therapy [6] for other nonlabeled uses.[5] The use of BTX-A for many facial cosmetic procedures has been described extensively in the literature.[66-72]

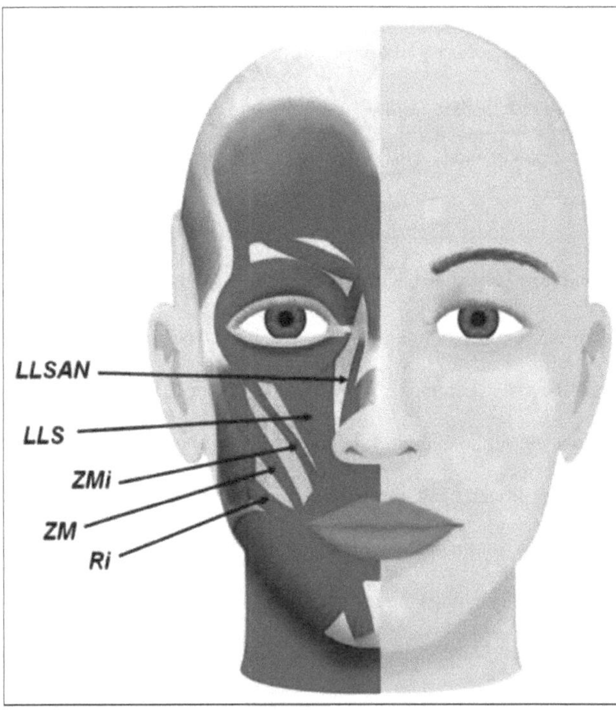

Fig.6.7.1 The Main muscles involved in gingival exposure are levator labii superioris alaeque nasi (LLSAN), levator labii superioris (LLS), zygomaticus minor (ZMi), zygomaticus major (ZM), and risorius (Ri).

Polo reported the benefits of BTX-A were reported in 5 patients with gummy smiles.[73]

The purpose of that pilot study was to determine whether injecting BTX-A at particular muscle sites could provide an alternative therapy for gummy smiles caused by hypercontractibility or excessive muscle contraction. The results were encouraging. The objective of this investigation was to determine whether the doses and the primary injection sites used in the pilot study for the correction of gummy smiles provide consistent, statistically significant, and esthetically pleasing results. A diversified group of health care professionals involved in various cosmetic treatments also served as evaluators. The goal was to identify a consistent, minimally invasive alternative for the correction of gummy smiles caused by hyperfunctional upper lip elevator muscles.

In later in 2008, a study was conducted by Mario Polo,[74] in which twelve women with excessive gingival display were injected at two sites with 1.25 U of botulinum toxin in the right and left levator labii superioris alaeque nasi muscles, and the overlap areas of the levator labii superioris and zygomaticus minor muscles. These injection were repeated in a second phase of the study one month later and followed by a 2.5 U injection in a third phase. Those that had the greatest amount of elevation near the philthrum also received injections at the origin of the depressor septi nasi muscle at the orbicularis oris muscle at each phase of the study. He found that all patients demonstrated improvement 10 days post-injection, while the maximum effect was observed 14 days post-injection with a mean decrease in gingival display of 4.2 mm. This effect was reversible, lasting for 3 to 6 months. He reports that all patients were pleased with the results and no side effects were reported or observed.[73]

In a follow up study by Polo to determine whether the dose and injection sites used in the pilot study produce consistent, esthetically pleasing results, Polo injected 30 patients with 2.5 U at the same sites as discussed in his pilot study and followed them at 2, 4, 8, 12, 16, 20 and 24 weeks post-injection with changes documented by photographs and videos. Again the maximum effect was observed at 2 weeks post-injection with a mean decrease in gingival display of 5.1 mm. The gingival display increased gradually, although the gingival display had not yet returned to baseline by week 24. It was estimated with a polynomial equation that the pre-treatment gingival display would not be reached until 30 to 32 weeks post-injection. At week 2, patients and a panel of specialty evaluators rated the effects of the botox injections via pre and post treatment photographs and videos on a 1 to 5 point scale with 1 representing poor and 5 representing excellent. Both patients and specialists rated the results between very good and excellent with a mean of 4.66 and 4.65 respectively.[74]

In a letter to the editor in response to Polo's article, Niamtu, relates experiences of unesthetic perioral animation in his patients treated with botulium toxin injections. He states, "they looked dysfunctional," described a "range from slight change in smile, pucker, and word pronunciation to a "stroke like" expression in some phases of animation." He suggests that the photos in Polo's study cannot truly display the appearance of the patients in animation. While he relates years of experience with botox, he warns that dramatic undesirable results can be produced by inexperienced practitioners including severe drooling, inability to pucker, grossly asymmetric smiles, inability to annunciate words, and a stroke like appearance.[75]

6 Later in 2009, a study by Hwang et. al., 4 the distribution, morphology, and direction of muscles fibers of the levator labi superioris (LLS), the levator labii superioris alaeque nasi (LLSAN), and the zygomaticus minor (ZMi) and major (ZMj) muscles

were examined in 25 adult and 34 cadavers with the aim of proposing a safe and reproducible injection point for botulinum toxin type A. They found that the three lip elevator muscles converged on the area lateral to the ala of the nose with no significant differences in the angular projection of the muscle fibers from origin to insertion between males and females or left side to right side. This area of convergence was prosposed as a safe and reproducible injection site for the botulinum toxin. The centre of this triangular area is known as the "Yonsei point".

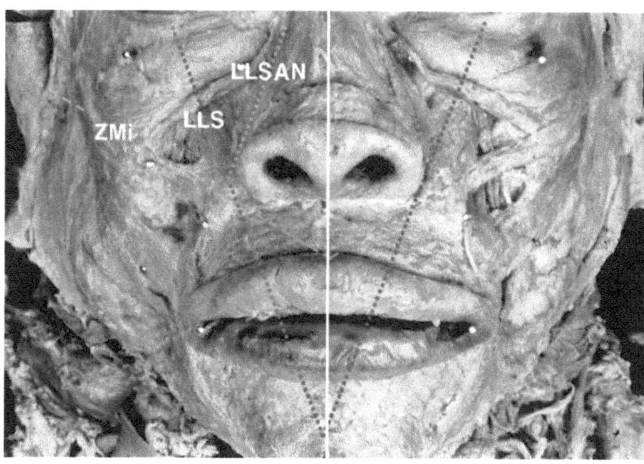

Fig.6.7.2

Fig.6.7.2Photograph of dissected specimen with vectors showing the direction of muscle fibers

Location of an Injection Point for BTX

Stainless steel pins were placed at the following surface landmarks before the dissection procedure was performed Fig.6.7.3.

1, 2: Lateral point of ala

3, 4: Midpoints of nasolabial fold between ala and commissure

5, 6: Maxillary point located at one-quarter distance between ala and tragus

7: Soft tissue subnasale

8, 9: Commissure

10: Soft tissue pogonion

11, 12: Lateral chin point located 2 cm lateral to pogonion (right and left) for standardization of measurement

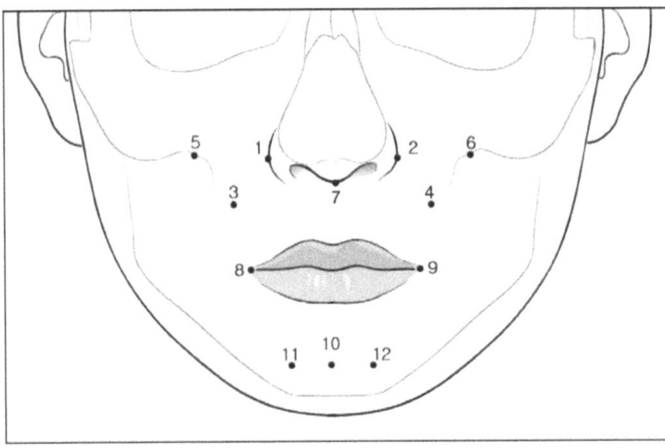

Fig.6.7.3 Surface landmarks used in this study

A triangular area was constructed by connecting the landmarks 1(2), 3(4), and 5(6) on each side (Fig.6.7.3). The effective range of BTX in this study was set at approximately 2 cm, as suggested by Garcia and Fulton Fig.6.7.5 Circles with a radius of 1 cm from each point and from the center of the triangle were drawn. The frequency of overlap with each muscle vector and the circular area from each landmark were counted under the assumption that a single injection of BTX at that point should affect all three muscles.

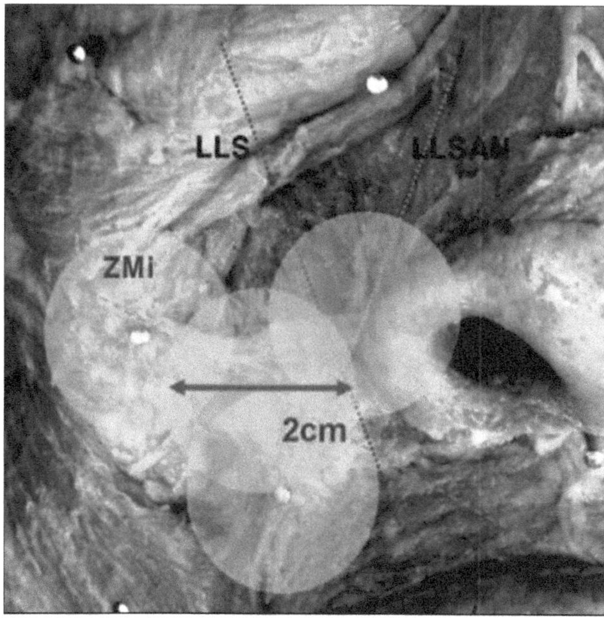

Fig.6.7.5 Circles with a 1 cm radius (2 cm diameter) drawn on each photograph represent the effective range of botulinum toxin.

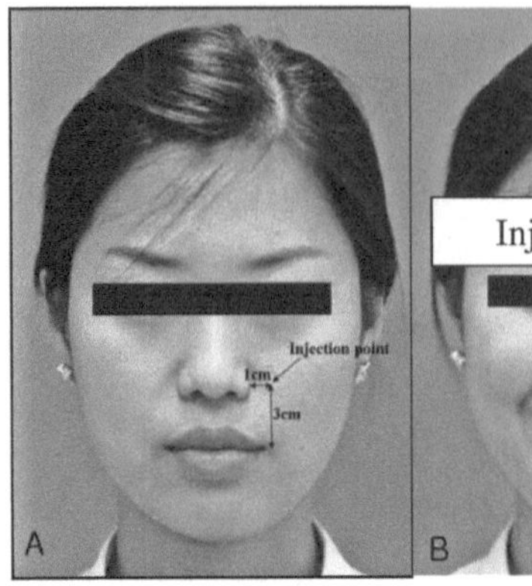

Injection point

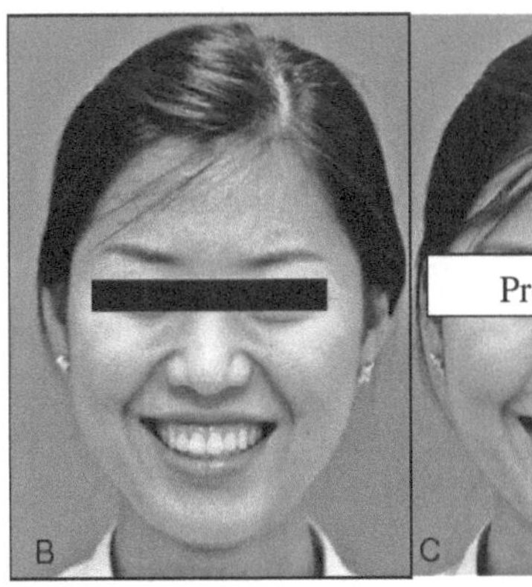

Pre-operative

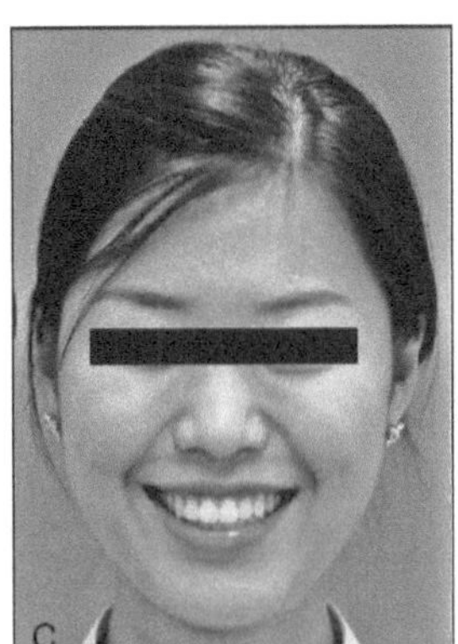

Post-operative

Fig.6.7.6 A-C

Injection at this site was demonstrated to be clinically effective in the reduction of a gingival smile due to muscular hyperfunction in two cases. [76] (Fig.6.7.6)

To summarize, while still in its early stages, literature and studies advocate use of botulium toxin type A and that it might be an effective, yet transient treatment for excessive gingival display.

SUMMARY

Excessive gingival display is an esthetic concern both to the patient and the clinician, especially when restoration of the anterior teeth is indicated. Understanding the etiology and treatment modalities is crucial in the process of treatment of a patient with a gummy smile.

Consequently, along with the knowledge to treat patients that present with "gummy" smiles, considerable emphasis should be given to recognize those that have a tendency to become "gummy," and to prevent the development of a "gummy" smile during orthodontic treatment.

There is agreement in defining gummy smile as a continuous band of gingival display of more than 3 mm, during spontaneous smile. The etiologic factors may occur alone or in combination. These include: skeletal problems (dental and bone); gingival disorders (passive eruption and gingival hyperplasia); and muscle problems (upper lip length and muscular hyperactivity).

The biologic mechanism underlying the gingival smile line appears to include the combined effects of several variables :

1. Anterior vertical maxillary excess (2 – 3 mm additional)
2. Greater muscular capacity to raise the upper lip on smiling (≥1mm additional)
3. Supplemental associated factors, including excessive overjet, excessive interlabial gap at rest and excessive overbite.

Therapeutic alternatives, in accordance with the underlying etiology, are usually multidisciplinary and multifactorial. The following alternatives are presented in the literature:

- Periodontal surgery for cases of excessive gingival display or passive eruption;
- Surgery of the muscular tissue for cases of short upper lip
- Orthognathic surgery in cases of excessive vertical growth;
- Orthodontic mechanics associated with intrusive mini implants in cases of overbite with extrusion of upper anterior teeth,

  And additional periodontal surgery to remove excessive gingival tissue and bone volume, resulting from the applied mechanics;
- Use of Botox or surgery of the muscular tissue for cases of hypercontraction of elevator muscles of upper lip.

Inter-disciplinary treatment combines aesthetic and biological principles, as well as prosthetic and surgical techniques essential to the success of a patient's comprehensive treatment. This will elicit favorable result esthetically as well as functionally to the patient and the clinician.

CONCLUSION

Gingival topography is a complex interplay of the underlying bony architecture and the size, form and position of teeth. The concept of modern day dental aesthetics places equal impetus on the "White" and "Pink" components, and a balance of the two is an essential ingredient in smile designing. Subsequently, in treating gummy smile patients, the initial approach must be a complete diagnostic procedure that identifies the etio-anatomo-pathological causes. Often, tooth wear may be associated with one or more of the etiologic factors, and in such cases a comprehensive and multidisciplinary approach is mandatory.

Also establishing the distinction between active or passive altered eruptions is necessary, because as in the first case the surgery required both osteoplasty and ostectomy, whereas in the second case a gingivectomy may be sufficient.[77] Performing only a gingivectomy in areas of AAE would lead to failure of the treatment caused by reestablishment of the biologic width at the same position.[77] Some authors suggest that esthetic and prosthetic reference points should be used to outline the surgical incision and also guide the quantity of ostectomy through a surgical guide.[78] Often though, asymmetrical wear of incisal margins, consequent asynchronous and asymmetrical compensatory eruption, and frequent possibility of altered eruption are observed. Surgically exposing the CEJ position is important.

Orthodontic treatment aligns the teeth in their ideal positions, and, finally, the restorative phase is completed. Therefore, when performing surgery with a biological approach, the correct reference point is not determined by the surgical guide but by the CEJ. The surgical guide maybe used for the soft-tissue incision to transfer the information extracted from clinical and radiographic examinations and not from an esthetically or prosthetically guided stent.

The restorative approach includes cases with previous crowns in which the CEJ can no longer be located; there are malaligned teeth, and teeth with loss of periodontal attachment. In these situations the goal of the surgery is to lengthen the crown using esthetic and structural parameters such as the crown-root ratio, the periodontal status,[7] and the incisal margin position.[9] With this approach, where full-crown restorations are already present with margins apical to the CEJ, the emergence profiles are often over-contoured to promote biologically acceptable gingival contours, although this can lead to an esthetic compromise.[79]

Periodontists may adopt two different approaches when treating gummy smile and short tooth syndrome patients: biological or restorative. Regardless of the planned therapeutic approach, misdiagnosis of an altered eruption due to the absence of a valid and repeatable diagnostic protocol can create esthetic and periodontal failures, such as disproportioned teeth and unnatural lengthening of incisal margins, which may jeopardize the smile and facial esthetics and cause longer anterior guides.[80] Furthermore, restorative margins placed too far coronally from the CEJ may be at risk of subsequent and progressive resolution and compensation of the altered eruption with time and, ultimately, esthetic failure.

Owing to which use of an accurate diagnostic protocol, an adequate and often multidisciplinary treatment is sufficient to compensate for the alteration of pink/white morphology and create a more pleasing and harmonious smile, even without completely resolving the etiopathological causes.

REFERENCES

1) Tjan AH, Miller GD, The JG. Some esthetic factors in a smile. The Journal of prosthetic dentistry. 1984 Jan 1;51(1):24-8.

2) Silberberg N, Goldstein M, Smidt A. Excessive gingival display--etiology, diagnosis, and treatment modalities. Quintessence international. 2009 Nov 1;40(10).

3) Hong RK, Lim SM, Heo JM, Baek SH. Orthodontic treatment of gummy smile by maxillary total intrusion with a midpalatal absolute anchorage system. The Korean Journal of Orthodontics. 2013 Jun 1;43(3):147-58.

4) Simon Z, Rosenblatt A, Dorfman W. Eliminating a gummy smile with surgical lip repositioning. The Journal of Cosmetic Dentistry. 2007;23(1).

5) Suma T, Shashikumar HC, Lokesh NK. Arya S, Shweta GS. Orthodontic Surgical Treatment of Gummy Smile with Vertical Maxillary Excess. IOSR J Dent Med Sci. 2014;13(10):68-74.

6) 10) Oliveira MT, Molina GO, Furtado A, Ghizoni JS, Pereira JR. Gummy smile: A contemporary and multidisciplinary overview. Dental Hypotheses. 2013 Apr 1;4(2):55.

7) Mazzuco R, Hexsel D. Gummy smile and botulinum toxin: a new approach based on the gingival exposure area. Journal of the American Academy of Dermatology. 2010 Dec 31;63(6):1042-51.

8) Kim TW, Freitas BV. Orthodontic treatment of gummy smile by using mini-implants (Part I): Treatment of vertical growth of upper anterior dentoalveolar complex. Dental Press Journal of Orthodontics. 2010 Mar 1;15(2).

9) Wu H, Lin J, Zhou L, Bai D. Classification and craniofacial features of gummy smile in adolescents. Journal of Craniofacial Surgery. 2010 Sep 1;21(5):1474-9.

10) Garber DA, Salama MA. The aesthetic smile: diagnosis and treatment. Periodontology 2000. 1996 Jun 1;11(1):18-28.

11) Oliveira MT, Molina GO, Furtado A, Ghizoni JS, Pereira JR. Gummy smile: A contemporary and multidisciplinary overview. Dental Hypotheses. 2013 Apr 1;4(2):55.

12) Geron S, Atalia W. Influence of sex on the perception of oral and smile esthetics with different gingival display and incisal plane inclination. The Angle orthodontist. 2005 Sep;75(5):778-84.

13) Schendel SA, Eisenfeld J, Bell WH, Epker BN, Mishelevich DJ. The long face syndrome: vertical maxillary excess. American journal of orthodontics. 1976 Oct 1;70(4):398-408.

14) Waldrop TC. Gummy smiles: the challenge of gingival excess: prevalence and guidelines for clinical management. InSeminars in orthodontics 2008 Dec 31 (Vol. 14, No. 4, pp. 260-271). WB Saunders.

15) Newman MG, Takei H, Klokkevold PR, Carranza FA. Carranza's clinical periodontology. Elsevier health sciences; 2011 Feb 14.

16) Fields HW, Proffit WR, Nixon WL, Phillips C, Stanek ED. Facial pattern differences in long-faced children and adults. American journal of orthodontics. 1984 Mar 1;85(3):217-23.

17) Isaacson JR, ISAACSON RJ, SPEIDEL TM, WORMS FW. Extreme variation in vertical facial growth and associated variation in skeletal and dental relations. The Angle Orthodontist. 1971 Jul;41(3):219-29.

18) Peck S, Peck L, Kataja M. The gingival smile line. The Angle orthodontist. 1992 Jun;62(2):91-100.

19) Brundo GC. The kinetics of anterior tooth display. J prosthet Dent. 1978;39:502-4.

20) McNamara L, McNamara JA, Ackerman MB, Baccetti T. Hard-and soft-tissue contributions to the esthetics of the posed smile in growing patients seeking orthodontic treatment. American Journal of Orthodontics and Dentofacial Orthopedics. 2008 Apr 30;133(4):491-9.

21) Singer RE. A study of the morphologic, treatment, and esthetic aspects of gingival display. American Journal of Orthodontics. 1974 Apr 1;65(4):435-6.

22) Alpiste-Illueca F. Altered passive eruption (APE): a little-known clinical situation. Med Oral Patol Oral Cir Bucal. 2011 Jan 1;16(1):100-4.

23) Matthews TG, Blatterfein L, Morrow RM, Payne SH. The anatomy of a smile. The Journal of prosthetic dentistry. 1978 Feb 1;39(2):128-34.

24) Rakosi T, Jonas I, Graber TM. Orthodontic diagnosis. Thiene Medical Publishers Inc., 1993.

25) Cohen ES. Atlas of cosmetic and reconstructive periodontal surgery. PMPH-USA; 2007.

26) Zawawi KH, Malki GA, Al-Zahrani MS, Alkhiary YM. Effect of lip position and gingival display on smile and esthetics as perceived by college students with different educational backgrounds. Clinical, cosmetic and investigational dentistry. 2013;5:77.

27) Monaco A, Streni O, Chiara Marci M, Marzo G, Gatto R, Giannoni M. Gummy smile: clinical parameters useful for diagnosis and therapeutical approach. Journal of Clinical Pediatric Dentistry. 2005 Sep 1;29(1):19-25.

28) Bernimoulin JP, Lüscher B, Mühlemann HR. Coronally repositioned periodontal flap. Journal of Clinical Periodontology. 1975 Mar 1;2(1):1-3.

29) Cohen DW, Ross SE. The double papillae repositioned flap in periodontal therapy. Journal of periodontology. 1968 Mar;39(2):65-70.

30) Coslet JG. Diagnosis and classification of delayed passive eruption of the dentogingival junction in the adult. Alpha Omegan. 1977;70(3):24-8.

31) Garber DA. The edentulous ridge in fixed prosthodontics. Compend. Contin. Educ. Dent.. 1981;2:212-23.

32) Gottlow J, Nyman S, Karring T, Lindhe J. Treatment of localized gingival recessions with coronally displaced flaps and citric acid. Journal of clinical periodontology. 1986 Jan 1;13(1):57-63.

33) Langer B, Calagna L. The subepithelial connective tissue graft. The Journal of prosthetic dentistry. 1980 Oct 1;44(4):363-7.

34) Nabers JM. Free gingival grafts. Periodontics. 1966;4(5):243-5.

35) Pennel BM, Higgason JD, Towner JD, King KO, Fritz BD, Salder JF. Oblique rotated flap. Journal of Periodontology. 1965 Jul;36(4):305-9.

36) Sullivan HC, Atkins JH. Freeutogenous gingival grafts. 1. Principles of successful grafting. Periodontics. 1968 Feb;6(1):5.

37) Sullivan HC, Atkins JH. Free autogenous gingival grafts. 3. Utilization of grafts in the treatment of gingival recession. Periodontics. 1968 Aug;6(4):152-60.

38) Smukler H, Chaibi M. Periodontal and dental considerations in clinical crown extension: a rational basis for treatment. International Journal of Periodontics & Restorative Dentistry. 1997 Oct 1;17(5).

39) Celar AG, Freudenthaler JW, C˘elar RM, Jonke E, Schneider BA. The denture frame analysis: an additional diagnostic tool. The European Journal of Orthodontics. 1998 Oct 1;20(5):579-87.

40) Pandurić DG, Blašković M, Brozović J, Sušić M. Surgical treatment of excessive gingival display using lip repositioning technique and laser gingivectomy as an alternative to orthognathic surgery. Journal of Oral and Maxillofacial Surgery. 2014 Feb 28;72(2):404-e1.

41) Peck S, Peck L, Kataja M. Some vertical lineaments of lip position. American Journal of Orthodontics and Dentofacial Orthopedics. 1992 Jun 1;101(6):519-24.

42) Storrer CL, Valverde FK, Santos FR, Deliberador TM. Treatment of gummy smile: Gingival recontouring with the containment of the elevator muscle of the upper lip and wing of nose. A surgery innovation technique. Journal of Indian Society of Periodontology. 2014 Sep;18(5):656.

43) Ezquerra F, Berrazueta MJ, Ruiz-Capillas A, Arregui JS. New approach to the gummy smile. Plastic and reconstructive surgery. 1999 Sep 1;104(4):1143-50.

44) Robbins JW. Differential diagnosis and treatment ofexcess gingival display. Practical Periodontics and Aesthetic Dentistry 1999;11:265-272, quiz 273.

45) Jorgensen MG, Nowzari H. Aesthetic crown lengthening. Periodontology Ø00. 2001 Oct 1;27(1):45-58.

46) Jorgensen MG, Nowzari H. Aesthetic crown lengthening. Periodontology Ø00. 2001 Oct 1;27(1):45-58.

47) Ravon NA, Handelsman M, Levine D. Multidisciplinary care: periodontal aspects to treatment planning the anterior esthetic zone. Journal of the California Dental Association. 2008 Aug;36(8):575-84.

48) Levine RA, McGuire M. The diagnosis and treatment of the gummy smile. Compendium of continuing education in dentistry (Jamesburg, NJ: 1995). 1997 Aug;18(8):757-62.

49) Kao RT, Dault S, Frangadakis K, Salehieh JJ. Esthetic crown lengthening: appropriate diagnosis for achieving gingival balance. Journal of the California Dental Association. 2008 Mar;36(3):187-91.

50) Polo M. Botulinum toxin type A (Botox) for the neuromuscular correction of excessive gingival display on smiling (gummy smile). American journal of orthodontics and dentofacial orthopedics. 2008 Feb 29;133(2):195-203.

51) Simon Z, Rosenblatt A, Dorfman W. Eliminating a gummy smile with surgical lip repositioning. The Journal of Cosmetic Dentistry. 2007;23(1).

52) Miskinyar SA. A new method for correcting a gummy smile. Plastic and reconstructive surgery. 1983 Sep 1;72(3):397-400.

53) Rubinstein A, Kostianovsky A. Cosmetic surgery for the malformation of the laugh: Original technique. Prensa Med Argent. 1973;60:952.

54) Rosenblatt A, Simon Z. Lip repositioning for reduction of excessive gingival display: a clinical report. International Journal of Periodontics & Restorative Dentistry. 2006 Oct 1;26(5).

55) Litton C, Fournier P. Simple surgical correction of the gummy smile. Plastic and reconstructive surgery. 1979 Mar 1;63(3):372-3.

56) Polo M. Re:'Treatment of gummy smile: Nasal septum dysplasia as etiologic factor and therapeutic target'. Journal of Plastic, Reconstructive & Aesthetic Surgery. 2015 Oct 31;68(10):1344-5.

57) Ellenbogen R, Swara N. The improvement of the gummy smile using the implant spacer technique. Annals of plastic surgery. 1984 Jan 1;12(1):16-24.

58) Creekmore TD. The possibility of skeletal anchorage. J ClinOrthod. 983;17:266-9.

59) Kanomi R. Mini-implant for orthodontic anchorage. J clinOrthod. 997;31:763-7.

60) Ohnishi H, Yagi T, Yasuda Y, Takada K. A mini-implant for orthodontic anchorage in a deep overbite case. The Angle Orthodontist. 2005 May;75(3):444-52.

61) Carrillo R, Rossouw PE, Franco PF, Opperman LA, Buschang PH. Intrusion of multiradicular teeth and related root resorption with mini-screw implant anchorage: a radiographic evaluation. American Journal of Orthodontics and Dentofacial Orthopedics. 2007 Nov 30;132(5):647-55.

62) Ohmae M, Saito S, Morohashi T, Seki K, Qu H, Kanomi R, Yamasaki KI, Okano T, Yamada S, Shibasaki Y. A clinical and histological evaluation of titanium mini-implants as anchors for orthodontic intrusion in the beagle dog. American Journal of Orthodontics and Dentofacial Orthopedics. 2001 May 31;119(5):489-97.

63) Brin MF, Hallett M, Jankovic J, editors. Scientific and therapeutic aspects of botulinum toxin. Lippincott Williams & Wilkins; 2002.

64) Benedetto AV. The cosmetic uses of botulinum toxin type A. International journal of dermatology. 1999 Sep 1;38(9):641-55.

65) Binder WJ, Blitzer A, Brin MF. Treatment of hyperfunctional lines of the face with botulinum toxin A. Dermatologic surgery. 1998 Nov 1;24(11):1198-205.

66) Ward AB, Barnes MP, editors. Clinical uses of botulinum toxins. Cambridge University Press; 2007 Mar 22.

67) Kane MA. The effect of botulinum toxin injections on the nasolabial fold. Plastic and reconstructive surgery. 2003 Oct 1;112(5):66S-72S.

68) Carruthers J, Carruthers A. Botulinum toxin A in the mid and lower face and neck. Dermatologic clinics. 2004 Apr 30;22(2):151-8.

69) Keen M, Blitzer A, Aviv J, Binder W, Prystowsky J, Smith H, Brin M. Botulinum toxin A for hyperkinetic facial lines: results of a double-blind, placebo-controlled study. Plastic and reconstructive surgery. 1994 Jul 1;94(1):94-9.

70) Niamtu J. Aesthetic uses of botulinum toxin A. Journal of oral and maxillofacial surgery. 1999 Oct 1;57(10):1228-33.

71) Fagien S. Botox for the treatment of dynamic and hyperkinetic facial lines and furrows: adjunctive use in facial aesthetic surgery. Plastic and reconstructive surgery. 1999 Feb 1;103(2):701-13.

72) Rohrich RJ, Janis JE. Botulinum toxin type a: once feared, now revered. Plastic and reconstructive surgery. 2003 Feb 1;111(2):867-8.

73) Spósito MM. New indications for botulinum toxin type A in treating facial wrinkles of the mouth and neck. Aesthetic plastic surgery. 2002 Mar 21;26(2):89-98.

74) Polo M. Botulinum toxin type A in the treatment of excessive gingival display. American journal of orthodontics and dentofacial orthopedics. 2005 Feb 28;127(2):214-8.

75) Polo M. Botulinum toxin type A (Botox) for the neuromuscular correction of excessive gingival display on smiling (gummy smile). American journal of orthodontics and dentofacial orthopedics. 2008 Feb 29;133(2):195-203.

76) Niamtu J. Botox injections for gummy smiles. American Journal of Orthodontics and Dentofacial Orthopedics. 2008 Jun 30;133(6):782-3.

77) Hwang WS, Hur MS, Hu KS, Song WC, Koh KS, Baik HS, Kim ST, Kim HJ, Lee KJ. Surface anatomy of the lip elevator muscles for the treatment of gummy smile using botulinum toxin. The Angle orthodontist. 2009 Jan;79(1):70-7.

78) Kim SJ, Kim JW, Choi TH, Lee KJ. Combined use of miniscrews and continuous arch for intrusive root movement of incisors in Class II division 2 with gummy smile. The Angle Orthodontist. 2014 Feb 7;84(5):910-8.

79) Van der Geld P, Oosterveld P, Van Heck G, Kuijpers-Jagtman AM. Smile attractiveness: self-perception and influence on personality. The Angle Orthodontist. 2007 Sep;77(5):759-65.

80) Hata K, Arai K. Dimensional analyses of frontal posed smile attractiveness in Japanese female patients. The Angle Orthodontist. 2015 Sep 14;86(1):127-34.

81) Dindaroğlu F, Duran GS, Görgülü S, Yetkiner E. Social smile reproducibility using 3-D stereophotogrammetry and reverse engineering technology. The Angle Orthodontist. 2016 May;86(3):448-55.

FSC
www.fsc.org
MIX
Papier | Fördert gute Waldnutzung
FSC® C083411

Kolibri 360 GmbH
Ferdinand-Jühlke-Straße 7
99095 Erfurt, Deutschland
produktsicherheit@kolibri360.de

Druck:
CPI Druckdienstleistungen GmbH
im Auftrag der
Kolibri 360 GmbH
Ferdinand-Jühlke-Str. 7
99095 Erfurt